BE YOU
DO YOU
FOR YOU

10 MINUTES ALL IN

Exercises for Seniors

CORE, BALANCE, AND BACK PAIN EXERCISES.

FULLY ILLUSTRATED GUIDE

for Weight Loss, Mobility and Mindfulness

(FROM BEGINNERS TO ADVANCED)

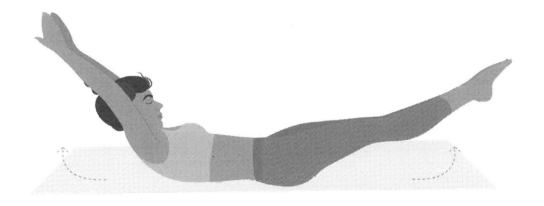

JONATHAN PRICE

JONATHAN PRICE

is an independent publisher, if you enjoy this book, please consider supporting us by leaving a review!

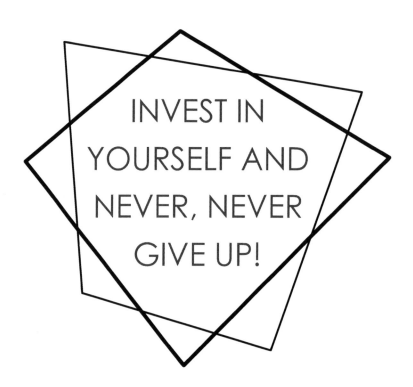

INVEST IN YOURSELF AND NEVER, NEVER GIVE UP!

THANK YOU FOR PURCHASING THIS BOOK,

IF YOU ENJOY THIS TITLE,

THEN FEEDBACK ON AMAZON WOULD BE

GREATLY APPRECIATED.

If you are not satisfied with this book, then drop us an email at:
selfcareemotional@gmail.com

We want our books to be truly enjoyable for everyone.

TABLE OF CONTENTS

Introduction

WHAT IS THE CORE? THE CORE IS THE CENTER OF OUR BODY, THE PROTECTIVE BOX OF OUR INTERNAL ORGANS. The front is made up of the rectus abdominis and the transverse muscles. The side walls are formed by the oblique abdominals. The posterior part is composed of the loins and spinal erectors. Finally, the bottom of the box is formed by the pelvic floor, and the lid by the diaphragm. All these muscles work in a coordinated way and it is important that the forces they exert are in balance with each other.

Before investigating further on the types of core stability exercises, it is essential to understand what this term means and what it is for.

From a purely scientific point of view, the term core stability identifies the ability of the respiratory diaphragm, the abdominal wall and the pelvic floor to stabilize the spine when any movement is made.

THIS TYPE OF TECHNIQUE IS INDICATED TO AVOID THE POTENTIAL ONSET OF INJURIES AND PAIN. We can therefore define it as an ideal way of acting and behaving to minimize problems related to sport and physical activity. An incorrect use of core stability leads to various problems in the back, which is particularly vulnerable and predisposed to degeneration in correspondence with impetuous and wrong movements.

WHEN WE APPROACH CORE STABILITY, WE REFER TO ALL THE MUSCLES OF THE ABDOMINAL-LUMBO-PELVIC COMPLEX, INCORPORATING A DOUBLE MUSCULATURE, THE DEEP ONE AND THE EXTERNAL ONE. In the first case, the muscles have the task of giving stability to the spine and pelvis, while in the second case the muscle band has the task of monitoring the movement of the limbs subject to gravity and external loads.

Wanting to give a simpler interpretation, we can say that the core is responsible for stabilizing the movement of the pelvis and thorax, favoring the expulsion of waste present in the muscles.

WHY IT IS IMPORTANT TO TRAIN THE CORE: ADVANTAGES AND BENEFITS

Core stability is of great importance in daily life as it brings with it various benefits. The main importance is found in the alleviation of back pain, that is all those problems related to the back of the body, particularly subject to the load of muscles and bones.

In order to have a clearer examination of the importance of core stability, it is essential to analyze the benefits individually. Specifically, concrete benefits are verified for:

- posture,
- lumbar problems,
- spine,
- knees and
- sports performance.

- IMPROVE POSTURE:

INCORRECT POSTURE SIGNIFICANTLY IMPAIRS THE RIGHT BALANCE BETWEEN BODY AND MIND. Postural pain and the consequences in the medium to long term can significantly affect people's health. Core stability allows you to fight incorrect posture and have the right postural behavior during the day. Many people underestimate the importance of correct posture, eventually finding themselves with very severe pain in the back and neck. Being able to better manage their posture over the years guarantees a healthier life physically, but above all it gives well-being to their psychological component. Through proper breathing, movement and muscle training, the body will automatically behave in the best way to protect the muscles.

- HELPS SOLVE LUMBAR PROBLEMS

LOWER BACK PAIN IS ONE OF THE MOST COMMON PROBLEMS IN PEOPLE WHO HAVE A SEDENTARY LIFESTYLE. About 90% of people suffer from this pathology at least once in their life, with inflammation to the point of inducing users to intervene with physiotherapy. One of the advantages of core stability is the concrete reduction of pain when suffering from lower back problems, guaranteeing a feeling of immediate relief with which to continue the working or sports day without any thought.

- VERTEBRAL COLUMN

WHEN YOU HAVE LUMBAR PROBLEMS, IT IS VERY LIKELY THAT OTHER AREAS OF THE BODY ARE ALSO AFFECTED, one of the most recurrent problems is that inherent to the spine. Having the wrong position during daily activities, or not having an adequate posture, can lead to scoliosis or lordosis, and that is certainly not pleasant. Core stability takes care to induce users to behave appropriately to minimize problems of this entity, freeing the subject from potential physiotherapy treatments and annoying back pains.

- KNEES

THANKS TO CORE STABILITY IT IS POSSIBLE TO ELIMINATE ALL DAMAGE RELATED TO THE KNEES. Many people, especially those of a certain age, after a lifetime of walking in the wrong way, run into severe pain in the knees. Although in many cases there is a deterioration of the cartilage due to age, in many others the pains are due to inappropriate posture. Prevention in this case is essential to feel good about your body.

- IMPROVE SPORTS PERFORMANCE

ONE OF THE BENEFITS THAT SHOULD NOT BE UNDERESTIMATED IS IN MAINTAINING SPORTING PERFORMANCE, DUE TO THE GRADUAL IMPROVEMENT OF FLEXIBILITY.

The muscles need specific training to ensure maximum performance, and core stability minimizes potential muscle injuries, offering the subject a more careful planning of his training.

Many athletes use core stability to improve their physical performance throughout the year.

WHAT ARE THE CORE MUSCLES?

It is necessary to describe two types of muscles, internal and external ones. As highlighted in the definition of core stability, these have different functions.

AS FOR THE INTERNAL MUSCLES, those that belong to the core are: diaphragm, pelvic muscles, multifidus muscle, internal obliques and transverse abdominal muscle.

THE EXTERNAL MUSCLES involved are: quadrate loin muscle, erector spine muscle, external oblique muscles and rectus abdominis muscle.

THE MUSCLES IN THIS CASE ARE ESSENTIAL TO MOVE SAFELY AND ALWAYS HAVE CORRECT POSTURE. When imbalances arise, it is essential to have muscles ready to rebalance internal and external forces, so as not to create friction or injury to the most important parts of the body.

Having analyzed the theory, including the purpose and the reference muscles, one of the best conditions to understand the potential of core stability is to take a look at the best exercises to perform.

- PLANK

THE PLANK, AN ISOMETRIC ACTIVITY THAT COMBINES STRENGTH AND ENDURANCE IN THE SHORT TERM. Although core stability is characterized by several exercises, this is considered the fundamental one since it guarantees the best results in an extremely short time.

It is essential to perform it in the best way to get the maximum result.

One of the most frequent questions which sportsmen ask themselves when they approach core stability, concerns the real usefulness it can have in sports. Most of the core stability exercises are isostatic, i.e. they are characterized by on-the-spot movements aimed at improving muscle strength and endurance. Although from a purely superficial point of view it may be thought that core stability is not suitable for movement sports such as running and football, in reality it can be very useful to reduce potential injuries.

As also highlighted in the advantages of core stability, these exercises allow you to reduce pain in the lower back, spine, knees and other areas of the body. This can also be very useful for footballers and runners who want to reduce this.

EXERCISES FOR THE ELDERLY

Isometric activity could you lead to think that there are exercises indicated only for those who want to improve strength and endurance, but in reality, there are many exercises aimed precisely at older people who want to strengthen their muscles and knees.

Specifically, the most suitable exercises are plyometric ones. These allow you to also integrate the multiplanar components and further strengthen the posture. In recent years, more and more elderly people rely on exercises of this kind to reduce back pain to a minimum, guaranteeing a more peaceful and less anxious daily life.

CORE STABILITY EXERCISES FOR THE BACK

One of the most important back exercises is the crunch. By lying on your back, you can bend your legs and improve the endurance and strength of the abdomen. This exercise is usually combined with the lifting of the legs and arms with the torso resting on the mat. The extension of the muscle bands allows to significantly reduce back pain.

Raising the pelvis while lying on the mat also significantly helps your back, offering immediate relief when done with correct timing and without quick jerking.

Certainly, exercises such as the plank and crunches are indispensable in a training program, but many times it is more important to evaluate the cases individually to speed up the desired progress.

- MISTAKES TO AVOID DURING TRAINING

In an ideal training program, in addition to the exercises to be performed, it is essential to know the mistakes to avoid. An exercise performed poorly can involve more problems than an exercise aimed at a muscle band that you do not want to improve, but what are the errors to be ruled out during physical activity?

STRETCHING: one of the most common mistakes of those who practice physical activity is to skip stretching completely. Although the exercises that will be performed also have the function of awakening the muscles and internal organs, it is advisable to carry out stretching in order not to incur injuries due to the cold or sudden movements.

SPEED OF EXECUTION: many people, taken by the desire to reduce back pain, perform the exercises too quickly. The success of an exercise, especially for core stability, is through the perfect execution of the movements.

Slow moving is definitely a better condition for the awakening muscles, which can be speeded up when fully active.

ACCESSORIES TO USE: some core exercises take advantage of dedicated accessories to allow a better execution of the movement. Although there are many accessories on the market to help athletes, it is very important to know how to choose them.

An accessory that is disproportionate in weight and functionality can lead to more problems than solutions, invalidating a job that must be performed correctly in order not to inflame the muscle groups.

CORE STRENGTH: WHAT IS THE LINK WITH CORE STABILITY?

When discussing core stability, it is also easy to find the term core strength, but what does it mean and what connects them?

To understand the connection between these two terms it is appropriate to give a definition of core strength. This term identifies the center of gravity of the human body as the core, considering it the fulcrum and core of stability.

Many people associate this word with the abdominals, but in reality, it would be more suitable to consider it as the union of the muscles of the shoulders up to the pelvis. Everything related to movement, in this case, is considered the center of the core, then other muscles are inserted with respect to core stability.

SPECIFICALLY, THERE IS A CONTRAST BETWEEN THE MUSCLES OF THE ANTERO VERSION AND THOSE OF THE RETROVERSION, affecting the postural balance between them. What links core stability and core strength is muscle improvement and back pain reduction. Although we have a core positioned differently, the principle of balance between the muscles is very similar.

The core strength bases its philosophy on training that does not necessarily have to strengthen the core muscles, but aims at developing their reactivity. The two types of approach help individuals to significantly reduce pain, even if using two different approaches. The core exercises, whether aimed at stability or flexibility, is essential to prevent injuries and guarantee the muscles a natural evolution.

WHAT CORE TRAINING IS AND WHAT IT CONSISTS OF

THE STATIC AND DYNAMIC EFFECTIVENESS AND EFFICIENCY OF THE HUMAN BODY DEPEND ON CORE TRAINING. It includes the abdominal muscles (rectus abdominis, obliques and transverse), the paraspinal muscles, the quadrate of the loins, the muscles of the pelvic floor, buttocks and hip flexors. Core training is therefore the training of this part of the body, which, in order to be effective, must contain a mix of strength, flexibility and control.

Core training must therefore be functional to movement, for those who run, for example. The goal is to create unstable situations in which our core reacts, restoring balance.

You can perform static exercises, called isometric, or in movement, using your body, or small tools, to also improve the ability to balance. Ensuring a strong, stable and flexible core is the best way to achieve both performance results, such as running faster and more effectively, and aesthetic results.

Why Is It Important to Train the Core for The Elderly?

As we age, bones weaken, muscle mass and body flexibility decrease, and balance suffers. All these factors combined can lead to normal daily activities with less agility and, in the worst cases, to unexpected and dangerous falls.

To avoid such events as much as possible, it is important to train regularly, in order to keep your physique strong and dynamic.

A decisive role in avoiding falls would be played in particular by the core, that is the central part of the body between the lower portion of the torso and the lower edge of the pelvis.

To keep it in shape, there are specific exercises that are easy to do at all ages.

WHY IT IS IMPORTANT TO TRAIN THE CORE

Continuing to have a strong core even when you are no longer very young is important because this muscle group, representing the connection point between the upper and lower body, is responsible for most of the movements necessary to lead a satisfying life.

Training it is therefore a priority, which amplifies even more after the age of 50, because it is at that age that the body begins to weaken, making a more incisive contrasting action necessary.

In addition to preventing injuries, a stronger midsection helps improve body stability and coordination, counteract back pain, improve posture and daily movements.

However, limiting ourselves to this is not enough. To keep fit as the years go by, it's also important to add at least 10 minutes of moderate aerobic activity a day to your fitness routine. Ideal is walking or, if you have knee problems, cycling or swimming, which allow you to move without burdening the joints.

THESE ARE THE MOST SUITABLE EXERCISES TO STRENGTHEN THE CORE FOR OLDER PEOPLE.

Mobility also worsens with age.

Twists or Seated Twists

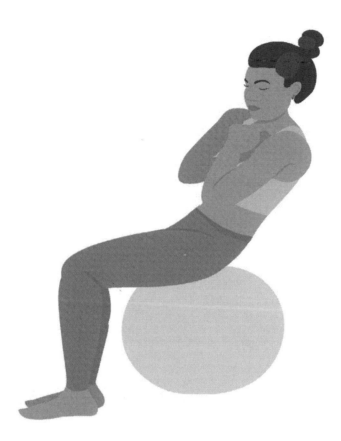

- Sit on an exercise ball and place your feet firmly on the ground in front of you.
- Bring your arms to your chest and lean back as comfortably as possible.
- As you engage your core muscles, rotate your torso to the left.

- Return to the starting position and repeat the sequence of movements on the right side.
- Complete three sets of fifteen reps each.
- If you can't reach that number, stop before the effort becomes too much.

Seated Knee Lifts

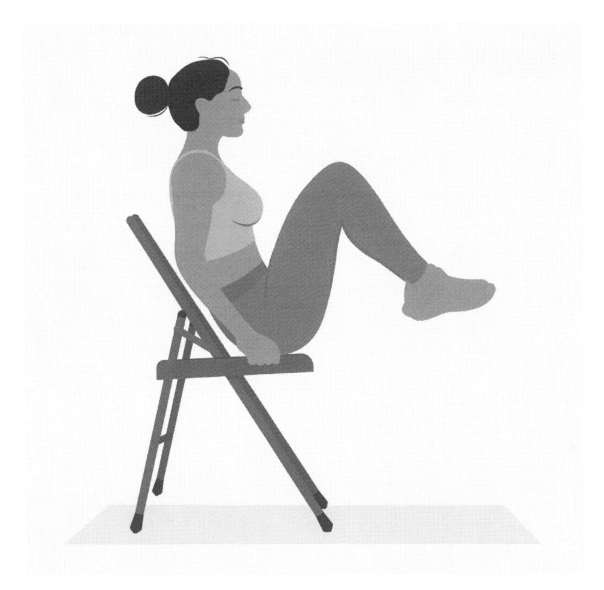

- Sit on a mat on the floor or, if you can't, on a bench.
- Move slowly and bring both knees towards your chest, trying to touch your abs with your legs.

- Use your hands if you feel you can't stay balanced.
- Return to the starting position.
- Perform three sets of fifteen repetitions each.

Kneeling Back Leg Raise

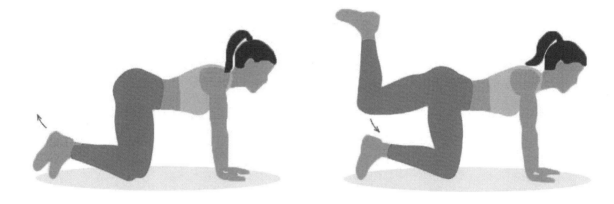

- Get on all fours, on your hands and knees and making sure your weight is evenly distributed on all four points.
- Extend your right leg back so it rises slightly above the ground.
- Keeping your leg straight, lift it as high as possible without arching your back or feeling pain. Lower it and return to the starting position.
- Repeat the sequence of movements on the other side.
- Perform three sets of ten repetitions each.

Glute Bridge

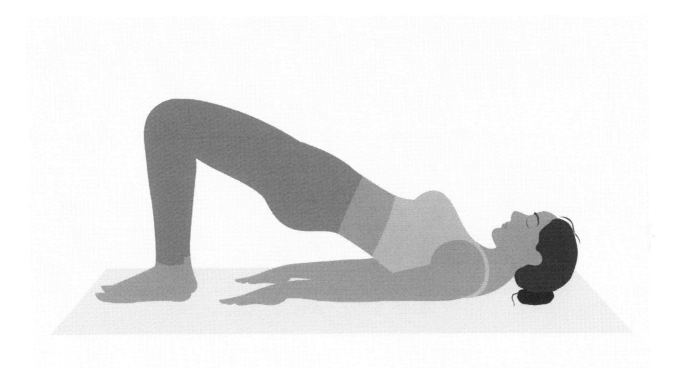

- Lie on your back with your knees bent and your feet flat on the floor, positioned hip-width apart.
- Push your lower back into the ground and contract your abdominal muscles.
- As you exhale, lift your hips off the floor until you form a diagonal line from the knees to the rib cage.
- Do not over-stretch your hips, to avoid damaging your lower back. Press your heels to the floor to keep yourself stable.
- Inhale and return to the starting position.
- Perform ten repetitions.

Curl Reclining

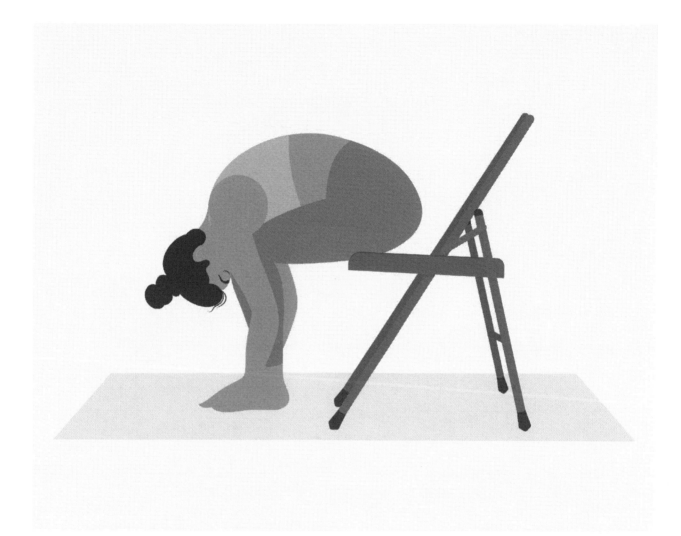

- Sit on a chair or bench, placing your feet firmly on the ground and contract your core muscles and abdominals for at least one minute.
- Keep the spine straight while inhaling and bringing the head back.

- Stop just before touching the backrest, exhaling as you return to the starting position.
- Perform two sets of five repetitions each.

Half Lunges

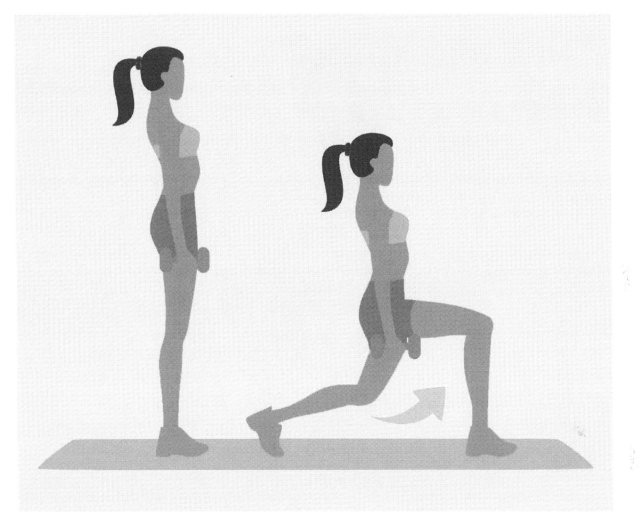

- Stand upright, keeping your feet together and your arms at your sides.
- Step forward and bend your left leg to form a right angle.
- Return to the starting position and repeat the same movement on the other side.

- Distribute your body weight evenly between the right and left foot.
- Do three sets of ten repetitions each.

Half Squats

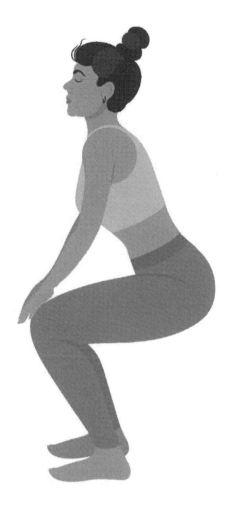

- Stand upright, with legs apart, feet turned slightly outward and hands resting on thighs.
- Bend your knees slightly while keeping your back straight.
- Stop before the buttocks reach the level of the knees.
- Exhale as you return to the starting position.
- Perform three sets of ten repetitions each.
- Do not lift your heels off the ground, and contract the abdominal and buttock muscles.

When we talk about core stability, we often only think of the abdominal muscles. However, the core includes not only the abs but also the lower back and hips.

The core is the body's center of gravity, and the stronger it is, the better we will be able to move, both when exercising and in everyday movements.

IN FACT, HAVING A TRAINED CORE MEANS:

- improved stability of the body
- improved coordination
- reduced risk of injury
- help counteract back pain
- improved posture
- improved daily movements

CORE STABILITY EXERCISES MUST PROGRESS FROM A BASIC LEVEL TO GREATER DIFFICULTY. We will start from the acquisition of basic motor skills. We will then move on to a functional progression, to reach the phase in which activation will become automatic and can be integrated into sport-specific activities.

The initial core stability exercises are performed on the floor, then you can progressively move to a less stable environment, so that the movements become more complex.

CORE TRAINING: WHAT IT IS, BENEFITS, EXERCISES AND STABILITY

The continuous progress in today's society is also reflected in the methods and concepts of training, both for professional sportsmen and for amateur athletes or ordinary people with a keen desire to keep fit.

This progress has led to improvements in knowledge regarding the usefulness of functional training, which has its roots in training and development of the core, together with the muscles that compose it. This is how core training was conceived!

WHAT IT IS AND FEATURES

In recent years, the concept of Core and more specifically Core Stability has been the subject of extensive discussions and scientific research.

The meaning of the term core is that of minscore or centermins, although to give a more precise idea of which muscles are considered part of the core - considering the incorrect concept of core which over time has spread according to which the muscles involved would be those of the abdomen and their reinforcement, was therefore considered sufficient - the NASM (National Academy of Sport Medicine) has given a meaning that leaves little room for interpretation.

THE UNION OF TWO MUSCLE CHAINS IS THEREFORE CONSIDERED CORE. The latter is formed by the stabilizer system and the movement system or better called minsglobal musculaturemins.

Both muscle chains have the task of generating and transferring forces from the trunk to the limbs and vice versa during the performance of numerous daily activities.

SPECIFICALLY, THE STABILIZER CHAIN INCLUDES THE FOLLOWING MUSCLES:

1. Transverse of the abdomen;
2. Internal oblique;
3. Transverse lumbar spinal;
4. Diaphragm.

INSTEAD, THE CHAIN OF MUSCLES THAT MAKE UP THE MOVEMENT SYSTEM INCLUDES:

1. Quadriceps;
2. Abdomen;
3. External oblique;
4. Square of the loin;
5. Gluteus maximus;
6. Spinal erector.

The union between these two muscle chains allows the stabilization of the body and the optimization of the motor scheme during the execution of the exercises or technical gestures.

At the same time, their training is fundamental for the prevention of musculoskeletal pathologies, in maintaining correct posture and the subsequent improvement of sports performance.

WHY TRAIN THE CORE?

Before listing a series of exercises and distribution of the workload that can be put into practice, it is a must to report the thought of authors and scholars, according to which the weakness of the core would be a determining factor behind many injuries.

A WEAK MUSCULATURE CAN AFFECT POSTURE, hindering the correct position of the hips / trunk and thus exposing the subject to a greater probability of incurring knee injuries.

Furthermore, POOR ACTIVITY OF THE PELVIS MUSCLES COULD LEAD TO A VARUS HIP (abnormal position of a part of the limb inwards) with consequent valgus in the knees (abnormal position of a part of the limb, this time outwards) due to stress induced by jumps or squats.

Furthermore, a below average level of core stability predisposes the subject to injuries to the ACL (anterior cruciate ligament).

On the contrary - let us remember - WORKING IN THE RIGHT WAY IN THE AFFECTED AREA IS A SOURCE OF MULTIPLE BENEFITS.

Among the first we remember THE PROGRESSIVE REDUCTION OF ANY POSTURAL IMBALANCES, the prevention of some pathologies affecting the skeleton, limbs and muscles, improvement of sports performance, with consequent optimization and improvement of the movements carried out in everyday life.

So, now that we have treated the core under different aspects, and having specified the benefits and above all the risks to which one is exposed in the absence of an underdevelopment of the muscle chains that compose it, let's continue with an overview of the composition of the work to be done, through some simple and targeted exercises.

CORE STABILITY WORK SETTING

As I have already explained to you, the development of the core and the muscular complex that composes it is important not only for those who practice sports.

In fact, the number of people who, regardless of age, approach this kind of functional training with the main aim of preventing or treating pathologies, which can arise due to the continuous stresses of which our body is a victim, is increasing every day.

Obviously, each person will need specific training based on the goal they are interested in achieving. There are several variations of exercises that are part of a core training program and include the current types of work:

- balance training;

- plyometric work;
- propioceptive exercises;
- joint stabilization movements;
- exercises that recall specific gestures for a specific sport.

USEFUL EXERCISES

Exercises can be performed both free body and with the help of objects such as kettle bells, proprioceptive tablets, swiss ball and medicine ball.

Bodyweight exercises can be performed isometrically, which then must be counterbalanced by other proprioceptive exercises.

Therefore, among the best exercises to perform to strengthen the affected area we find the plank, mountain climber, crunch, superman, exercises with the medicine ball.

PLANK

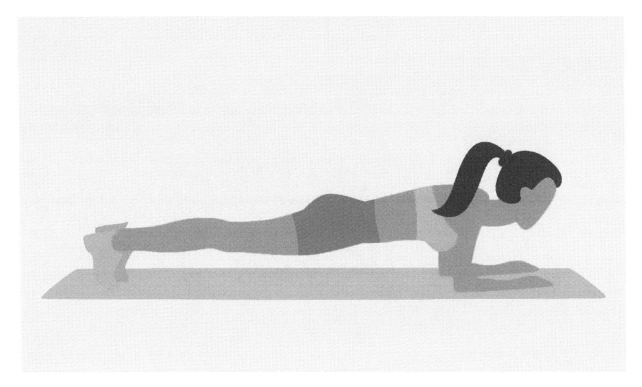

The plank is one of the most strenuous exercises to do mainly for abdominal strengthening, but at the same time it allows you to train almost all the muscles of the body.

You start lying down, with your stomach on the mat. Next, bend your elbows to 90 degrees making sure they are aligned with your shoulders.

Use as a support exclusively the forearms and toes, without the help of the hands.

Hold your hips high without twisting to try to maintain balance.

Contract the abdomen and try not to raise the pelvis too much, also do not bring the shoulders close to the ears. The gaze must be kept downward, so that the neck is not in tension.

Once this position has been reached, it must be maintained for as long as possible. There is no limit or an ideal time, but based on how long you can resist you can understand how much the core is more or less developed.

Below 30 seconds the core is underdeveloped; between 30 and 60 seconds the core is averagely developed; between 60 and 120 seconds, the core is well developed.

MOUNTAIN CLIMBER WITH BUST ROTATION

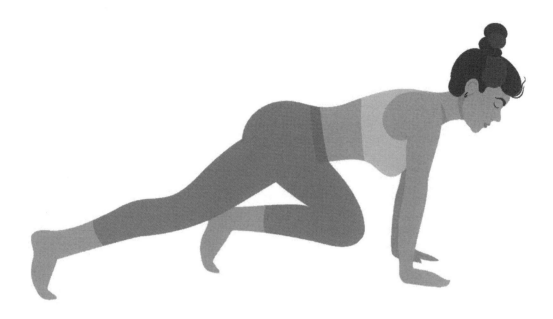

The starting position of the mountain climber with rotation is the same as for the plank, but with outstretched arms.

- From the starting position, start the exercise by moving the right knee in the direction of the opposite elbow;
- Once the knee is bent, make a slight rotation of the torso;
- As soon as you get to the end, stay in position for a second, making sure not to bring your shoulders close to your ears and to keep the line between shoulders, head and torso as much as possible;
- Bring the knee back by placing the foot on the ground again and repeat the whole movement on the left side.
- The mountain climber should be followed quickly with the help of a light jump, but those unfamiliar with the exercise are advised to proceed more slowly in order to avoid muscle tears.

REVERSE CRUNCH

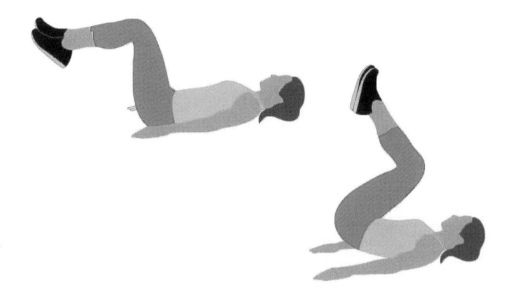

You will need the help of a yoga mat.

- Lie on the mat, bend your legs and make sure your feet are in contact with the floor;
- Keep arms stretched to the sides of the body;
- Begin the exercise by moving your knees towards your chest. The buttocks can rise but it is advisable to maintain stability and control of the legs, with the help of the hands and arms to avoid imbalances and injuries to the lumbar area;
- Especially when returning to the starting position, try to activate all the core muscles;
- Monitor the lower back by making sure that it remains in a neutral position;
- Finally, do not take your neck off the floor as you perform the exercise and make sure your shoulders are away from your ears.

SUPERMAN

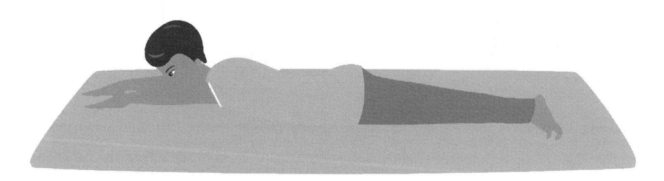

This exercise helps in toning the abdomen, but also the lower back. Here, too, you will need the help of a mat to best perform the superman exercise.

- Lie on the ground, with the belly down, the legs straight, the arms extended in front of the head and the palms facing the ground;
- Contracting the buttocks and lower back, lift the legs and upper body off the ground at the same time;
- Maintain the position for a few seconds and then slowly descend;
- Always make sure your neck is relaxed and your shoulders are away from your ears. If you feel tension in your lower back while exercising, stop moving.

What is Core Stability?

Core stability is a fundamental component for the physical well-being of each person and is created by the simultaneous and coordinated interaction of different muscles present right at the core level.

Talking about core stability is fundamental in many areas of the human body ranging from athletic training to rehabilitation, passing through postural and / or preventive adapted gymnastics.

Let's imagine having a balloon inside our belly and having to keep it stable in the center.

Having a stable abdomen also allows our whole body to be stable, as well as allowing limb movements to take place in a safer, more precise and coordinated way.

Let us immediately specify that we are not talking about the abdominal muscle group alone, but about the stabilizing local musculature and the one that makes up the movement system.

ITS FUNCTION

The system that includes all the muscles of the hips, back, abdomen, pelvis and diaphragm is fundamental for both static and dynamic balance.

This translates into greater stability and performance of the movement itself.

We can therefore define the core stability function as:

The ability of the body system to recover its equilibrium position at the level of the trunk, and beyond, after its external disturbance (rough ground for example).

The possibility of producing, transferring and controlling strength and motility in the legs and arms through the kinetic chains in the best way possible.

All the muscles in our body cannot work alone, but are connected with many others to perform their action in a synergistic way.

We are talking about muscle chains that run throughout our body, from the feet to the head: the core is the center, the central ring through which all these paths of movement pass, all these forces of contraction.

HOW TO TRAIN CORE STABILITY

We come to the reason why most of you have chosen to read this article, how to train in the best way to core stability.

The most important thing is the functional evaluation of the muscles that we have indicated above: in each person it is very easy to find very evident differences in terms of strength, contraction and shortening for each of them.

Having made this necessary clarification, let's see some useful exercises:

We inhale and exhale trying to inflate and deflate the belly and not the chest to activate the diaphragm muscle (correct breathing is the basis of core stability).

We inhale and then exhale forcibly until we have no more air to activate the transverse abdominis.

We activate the pelvic floor muscles as when we try to hold back the urge to urinate.

We work on the rectus abdominis and the obliques using the different types of crunches (please do not lift your legs, if not starting from 90 degrees and absolutely never before having trained your abdominals properly).

WE TRAIN THE BACK MUSCLES CAREFULLY.

Very useful are all those exercises in instability with the use of elastic bands, trx, proprioceptive discs, Bobath balls and other tools with which it is also possible to train the back muscles; just staying seated, for example, on proprioceptive discs or balls allows you to train the core muscles in a postural way (do not sit there 8 hours a day, though).

A typical exercise is the one that sees us prone, with only forearms and feet resting on the ground, with back and legs very straight and abdomen contracted (let's see how long you can maintain the position).

All other muscles related to movement must be tested first to know if they need to be strengthened or stretched.

Obviously, these are basic exercises that are easy to perform, but there are many other more complex and performing ones suitable for all needs.

POSTURE AND POSTURAL GYMNASTICS

The importance of posture in everyone's life is now a fact, and core stability is the basis of any type of postural gymnastics: working on the center of our body is the starting point to prevent injuries, improve chronic pain situations or even just working on your own body language.

Without precise and timely work on core stability, our postural training could be affected without allowing us to achieve the results we hoped for.

Once the abdomen has been stabilized, it will be possible to work on every aspect of posture in a safer, easier way as well as simpler training through other techniques that we will consider most appropriate (such as work on the kinetic chains).

Core stability: the basic exercises

If you really want to understand what it is, you have to consider the belly as the core and imagine keeping a very delicate object in balance right at that point. This takes on a deeper value than one can imagine: having a stable abdomen allows the whole body to be more precise and to move the limbs in a safer and more coordinated way. This does not mean that only the abdominal musculature should be taken into consideration: core stability focuses on the stabilizing musculature and on what constitutes the movement system.

Train core stability

What kind of exercises should you do to train core stability best? One of the most useful is undoubtedly the plank, followed by exercises that train the back (elastic, trx, Bobath ball or fitness ball, proprioceptive discs, etc.). Some types of breathing are also useful (inhaling and exhaling trying to inflate the belly instead of the chest, to activate the diaphragm) or pelvic floor stimulation (activating the muscles by emulating the contraction of the muscles that takes place when fending off urination). Finally, the classic crunch (supine, with the feet on the ground and the legs at 90°, bring the head to the knees avoiding touching the ground with the back) and the lateral crunch (same movement but working right arm and left leg, to then reverse and do the exact opposite).

- Prone plank
- Bird dog exercise
- Side plank

Prone plank

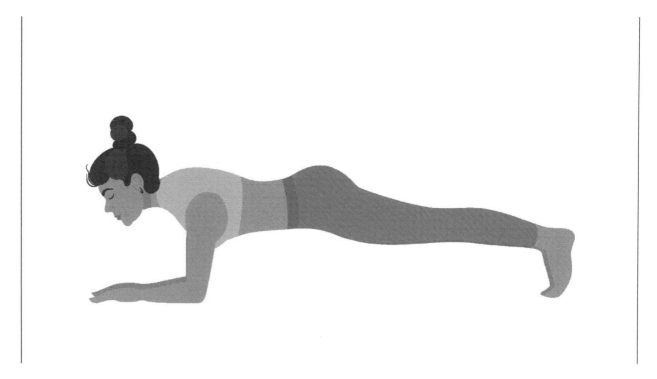

OBJECTIVE: development of core stability and strengthening of abdominal muscles and transverse muscle.

REPS: hold the position 30 seconds for beginners - 60 for experts.

SERIES: 3

REST BETWEEN SETS: 20 mins

DESCRIPTION:

- lie on your stomach, bending your elbows and leaning on the forearms on the floor.
- Keep the elbows in line behind the shoulders. Raise the chest and straighten the body until it forms a straight line from the head to the feet. Support the body and contract the abdominal muscles for the duration of the exercise.
- If the exercise is too strenuous, lean on knees instead of toes.
- To avoid onset of lower back pain, always keep the body aligned, avoiding holding the hips too high or too low.

Bird dog exercise

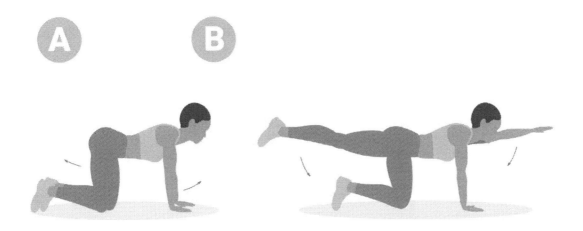

OBJECTIVE: to strengthen muscles of the spine, in especially the spinal erectors. Also, reinforcement of the buttocks, trapezius and deltoids.

REPS: 10 per side

SERIES: 3

REST BETWEEN SETS: 20 mins

DESCRIPTION:

- Start on your hands and knees with the hands under the shoulders and the knees under the hips. Slowly lift an arm forward, holding it by the side of the head, and simultaneously raise the opposite leg.
- Maintain the position for 3 seconds and then return to the starting one. Perform the movements slowly. The back must remain neutral; in final position, arm, back and leg must be aligned. To avoid rotation of the back that could cause low back pain, the leg raised must be parallel to the ground, and it must not go higher than the hip.
- The neck must to remain in a neutral position, it must not bend backwards or dangle forward.

Side plank

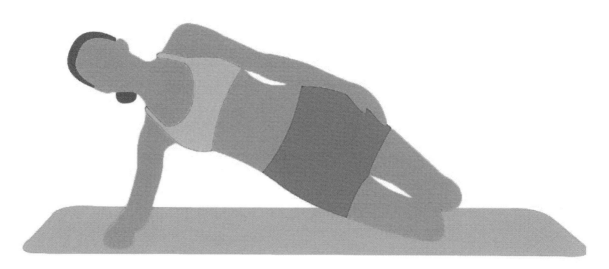

OBJECTIVE: strengthening of core stability and reinforcement of the abdominal muscles, especially muscle crosswise.

REPS: hold the position 30 mins for beginners - 60 mins for experts

SERIES: 3

REST BETWEEN SETS: 20 mins

DESCRIPTION:

- lie down on your side, touching the ground only with the outside of the leg and hip.
- The elbow is put below the shoulder and perpendicular to it, and the forearm is also placed on the ground, in front of the body. Contract the abdominal muscle sideways to lift the whole body off the ground.
- Maintain the position for the specified time, breathing normally. During the exercise do not rotate your back; be careful to keep one ideal line between shoulder, hip, knee and ankle, making sure that the pelvis never sinks.

To make the exercise more strenuous, hold the free arm upward, in line with the shoulder.

- Legs
- Squat
- Reverse lunge
- Supine bridge

Legs

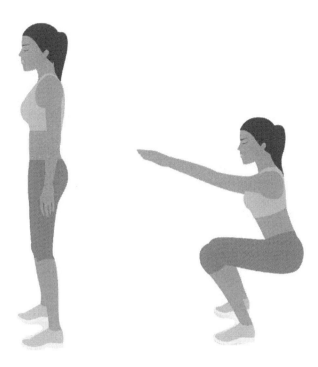

OBJECTIVE: to strengthen the muscles of the lower limbs, glutes, hamstrings and quadriceps, but also vertebral muscles and core stability.

REPS: 10 for beginners - 20 for experts

SERIES: 3

REST BETWEEN SETS: 20 mins

DESCRIPTION:

place your feet slightly more than shoulder wide with the toes slightly turned out.

Open the chest, keeping the shoulder blades relaxed. Look down slightly, like you're looking at an object a few meters ahead.

Slightly over-extend your back while pushing back the buttocks. At this point, holding the neutral back curvature, begin to descend, bending the knees. The ascent must take place maintaining the exact same set-up used in the descent. To perform the exercise safely, keep your back straight all the time and, during the descent, the knees must not project beyond your toes.

Squat

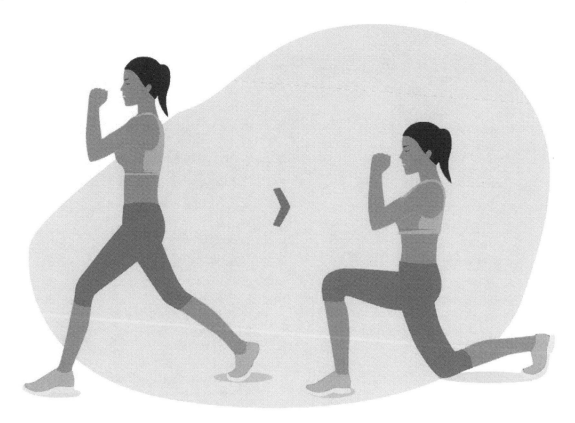

OBJECTIVE: strengthening of the lower limb muscles: glutes, hamstrings and quadriceps.

REPS: 10 for beginners - 20 for experts for side

SERIES: 3

REST BETWEEN SETS: 20 mins

DESCRIPTION:

Begin in a standing position and execute one step back. The knee of the leg that goes back must reach almost to the ground; the other leg must bend to 90°. Be careful not to misalign the pelvis during movement.

Reverse lunge

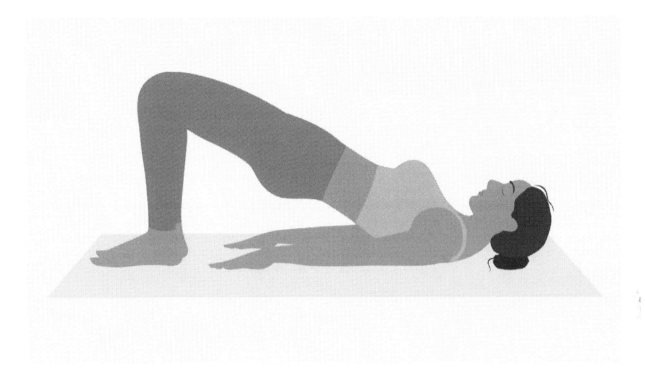

OBJECTIVE: reinforcement of the buttocks with the involvement of the extensor muscles of the hip (biceps femoral, semitendinosus and semimebranosus) and core.

REPS: 15 for beginners - 25 for experts

SERIES: 3

REST BETWEEN SETS: 20 mins

DESCRIPTION:

position yourself on your back, arms extended palms down, knees bent and heels close to the buttocks, about the width of the hips apart. By contracting the abdominal muscles, raise the pelvis from the ground by extending the hips, up to bringing the pelvis in line with the trunk and the femur. Do not go further, so as not to arch your back. Maintain the position for 3 seconds by contracting the buttocks.

Then return to the starting position restoring the lumbar area and then the sacral area.

Be careful not to arch your back in the step hip extension. Always keep your shoulders and the nape resting on the ground, without involving the cervical tract during exercise.

- ARMS for beginners
- Curl with elastic band
- Alternating hammer curl
- Bench dip
- Wall push off

ARMS for beginners

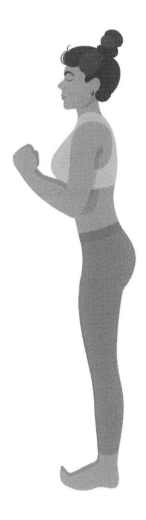

OBJECTIVE: to strengthen the muscles of the arms, especially the biceps.

REPS: 12

DESCRIPTION:

SERIES: 3

REST BETWEEN SETS: 90 secs

standing upright, with legs shoulder width apart and arms outstretched along the hips, slowly flex the forearm, keeping the elbow close to the body, and you return, always slowly, to the starting position.

Curl with elastic band

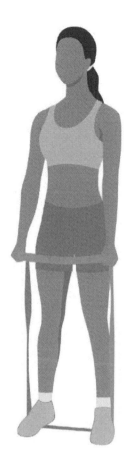
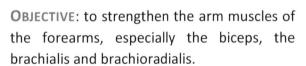
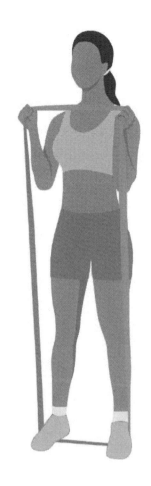

OBJECTIVE: to strengthen the arm muscles of the forearms, especially the biceps, the brachialis and brachioradialis.

REPS: 12

SERIES: 3

REST BETWEEN SETS: 90 secs

DESCRIPTION:

in a standing position, hold a set of dumbbells with neutral grip, i.e. with palms facing each other, and position yourself with feet shoulder-width apart. By contracting the abdominals, bring a dumbbell to the shoulder without changing the grip. Stop high, tighten the bicep, then slowly lower the weight to the starting position and repeat the gesture with the other arm.

Alternating hammer curl

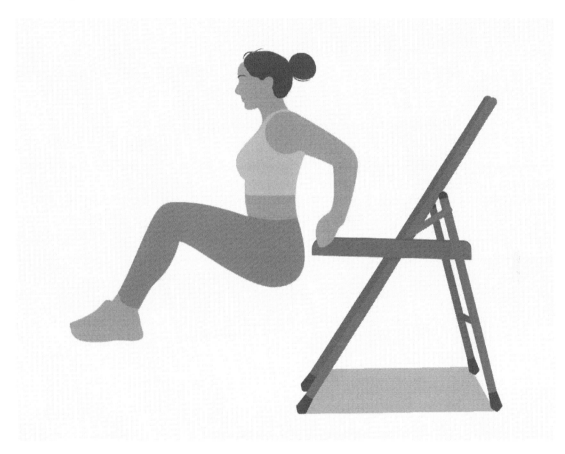

OBJECTIVE: to strengthen the muscles of the arms, especially the triceps.

REPS: 12-15

SERIES: 3

REST BETWEEN SETS: 90 secs

DESCRIPTION:

sit on the edge of a chair, place your hands on the seat, feet on the ground.

Push on your arms and bring your body forward with the buttocks suspended in the air. Bend the elbows to 90 degrees and drop the buttocks almost to the ground, then go back up with strength on your arms. The more you relax the legs, the harder the exercise, the more feet are near the chair or bench, the less difficulty.

Wall push off

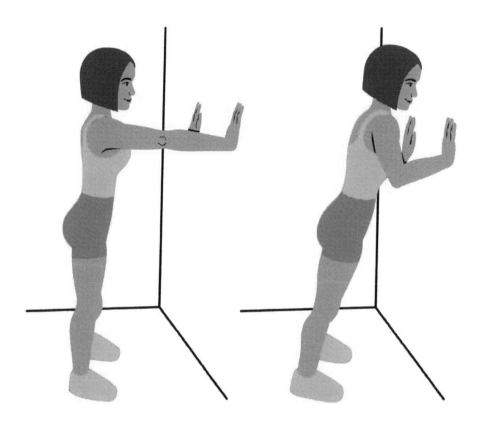

OBJECTIVE: to strengthen the muscles of the arms, especially the triceps.

REPS: 12

SERIES: 3

REST BETWEEN SETS: 90 secs

DESCRIPTION:

put your hands on the wall a little more than shoulder-width apart and take a step back with your feet so that your body is in a more stable position. Bend your elbows to bring your chest close to the wall, then push back so that your hands come off the wall and you lean over backwards on the toes. Then fall back towards the wall, bending the arms.

The abdominal muscles

First of all, it is necessary to mention the anatomy and the action of these muscles: in fact, the so-called abdominals are composed of four different muscles, which occupy the central cavity of the body and which act in synergy for flexion, torsion, rotation of the trunk and for the stability of the spine.

THEY ARE:

- Transverse abdominis
- Internal oblique
- External oblique
- Rectus abdominis

THE TRANSVERSE MUSCLES

It is the deepest of the abdominal muscles and acts by compressing the viscera, lowering the last six ribs and, in addition, recent studies have ascertained the importance of the correct timing of muscle contraction in stabilizing the lumbar area of the spine and in preventing lower back pain.

The tonicity of this muscle turns out to be really important, not only at a functional level, but also for those who aim only at aesthetic results, since the tonicity of the transversus allows a narrowing of the waist thanks to its function of containing the viscera: this can be achieved through special breathing exercises, such as the abdominal vacuum.

THE INTERNAL OBLIQUE

It is placed more internally than the external oblique and is involved in rotation and lateral flexion of the trunk.

It is inserted, with its posterior bundles, in the last three or four ribs, with its anterior bundles, at the height of the pectine crest and pubic tubercle and, with all its other bundles, in an aponeurosis which, splitting itself, goes to wrap the rectus abdominis.

THE EXTERNAL OBLIQUE

It is the largest of the abdominal muscles and is the most superficial of the four.

RECTUS ABDOMINUS

It is certainly the most discussed, it is a polygastric muscle characterized by transverse tendon inscriptions, clearly evident during contraction. Its action is fundamental for the flexion of the spine and also contributes in an important way to the rotation of the trunk.

It originates from the xiphoid process and from the 5th, 6th and 7th costal cartilage and is inserted, with a short and robust tendon, at the upper margin of the pubis, between the tubercle and the pubic symphysis. In the gym, users mistakenly believe that there are two types of rectus abdominis, the upper and the lower one, ignoring however that this is a single muscular belly that contracts mainly, flexing the spine and bringing the sternum closer to the pubis and vice versa.

WHAT ARE THE EXERCISES THAT MOST INVOLVE AND ACTIVATE THE ABDOMINALS?

Some research shows that, although of course there are no what are often improperly defined as high abdominals and low abdominals, nevertheless it is possible to define parts of the same muscle to give more emphasis to one region rather than another.

In fact, an interesting study that analyzed the EMG activation - the electrical activity of a muscle, i.e. the electromyographic analysis in this case of the abdominals - with the performance of 12 exercises, showed that the crunch with the hands facing the 'tall was the best exercise for hitting the upper region and hanging leg raises the best to hit the bottom more. Of course, it is impossible to completely isolate one area rather than another so during an exercise the entire muscular belly will work.

As for the obliques, it has been seen that the side bends and the total twisted crunch (hands to toes) are the best, therefore, since the action of the obliques is not only to tilt the torso sideways but also to rotate, the union of the two exercises, that is the twist with lateral inclination, could be the best possible training solution specific to that part.

Naturally, both the rotation movement and the inclination movement must be carried out slowly and in a super controlled way: especially during the torsion, you must never reach the position of maximum excursion because it can cause injuries to the lower back.

Exercises That Help to Get Up from The Ground

When a person is young, he can get up easily from the ground, without great effort or difficulty. However, as we age, this often becomes difficult. This is because as you get older, joint mobility, stability, and strength decrease. And as the joints become tighter and less stable and the muscles less strong, movement is more limited. The problem, however, is that on a normal day you have to get up (from the ground but simply also from a sitting position) and sit down many times a day, so if you lose your ability to do so, your quality of life takes a hard hit. In addition, the ability to get up from the ground is very important in the event of a fall, an event that becomes more common in old age. However, the loss of mobility and strength with age is not inevitable. There are strategies you can take to strengthen and stabilize your joints. One way is to incorporate specific exercises into your daily routine.

THE USEFUL LIFTING MOVEMENTS

As the name suggests, lifting exercises simulate the set of movements that take a person from sitting (or lying) on the floor to standing. The more you perform these types of movements, the more likely your joints are to remain trained and agile. You can start by doing the following variations of lifting exercises. They will help the practitioner transition gracefully from the floor to standing, improving strength, balance and coordination. It is advisable to repeat each

movement about ten times, even for several series if you want.

In addition to lifting exercises, it is helpful to do mobility movements to reduce the risk of developing tense, unstable and weak joints. A few minutes a day will suffice.

Supine Lying to Standing Get-Up

- Lie on your back with your arms at your sides and legs straight. Bend the right leg and bring it slightly out to the side, planting the right foot on the floor.
- Turn onto your left side, leaning on your left elbow.
- Straighten your left arm, applying force to your left hand and right foot to help swing your left leg under you, reaching a quadrupedal position on your hands and knees.
- Step forward with your right leg and raise your upper body to a semi-kneeling position.
- Press on both legs to rise to a standing position.
- Reverse the movements to return to the supine position.

This lifting exercise is critical because every human being must be able to master the transition from lying down to standing.

Crossed Legs Sitting to Standing Get-Up

- Sit cross-legged on the ground. Move the left leg back so that both knees are bent at an angle of approximately 45 degrees (the right foot will be in front of the left thigh, the left foot behind the buttocks).
- Push on both legs until you reach a kneeling position. If needed, you can use your hands for support.
- Step forward with your left foot and lift your upper body to a semi-kneeling position. Apply force on both legs to reach a standing position.
- Reverse the movements to return to the starting position.

This movement strengthens the mobility and stability of the hips.

Prone Lying to Standing Get-Up

- Lie on the ground on your stomach. Bend both elbows and bring your hands directly to your sides, with your palms on the ground.
- Press both hands to the ground and force on the arms by pushing towards the quadrupedal position on hands and knees. Step forward and raise your upper body to a semi-kneeling position.
- Apply force on both legs to reach a standing position and bring the feet together.
- Reverse the movements to return to the starting position.

How to Train For 10 Minutes A Day

If you are persistent and do the exercises well and with the right timing, you can get excellent results even by dedicating a few minutes a day.

WHAT CAN WE DO IN TEN MINUTES A DAY?

With ten minutes, then, you can do a workout for the complete abdomen, choosing an exercise every day to activate different muscle groups from time to time: from the rectus abdominis (the central muscle that starts from under the breastbone and reaches the pubis) to the oblique muscles, up to the transversus. One or two exercises of 3 or 4 series with 15/20 repetitions interspersed with one-minute breaks, or 40/45 for the most trained ones are enough.

HOW TO START THIS MINI-WORKOUT ON THE ABDOMEN?

What matters is choosing a good exercise that you can perform well and feel effective on your abdominal area. Many people, for example, have a bit of back stiffness or are unable to lift their legs. So, the first rule is to feel which exercise makes your abdomen work better.

HOW OFTEN IS IT BEST TO START?

I do not recommend full immersion from zero to one hundred for beginners. This training has to be approached gradually, because the body has to adapt. For those starting from scratch I recommend doing the exercises twice a week, then gradually going up to three, until stabilizing after a month to four times a week. And this is already a lot, because fitness training does not only include abs: let's not forget the rest!

I would like to point out immediately that with this abdominal work the adipose layer does not disappear. You will see an improvement in posture, tone and you will feel less back pain, but if you have inches of fat to lose, you must first focus on something else. The priority, in fact, for those who want to lose fat, is on the daily calorie deficit. By involving the abdomen and exerting end-abdominal pressure, it is recommended to do the exercises two hours after a meal, or on an empty stomach. Furthermore, as soon as you wake up your muscles are colder, while in the evening they are more flexible and with warm muscles it is better to train.

HERE ARE 4 EXERCISES TO DO WITH TEN MINUTES A DAY

The Crunch

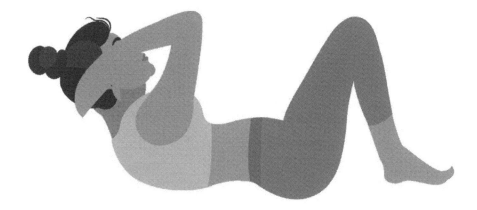

- Lying on your back with your legs bent at 45 degrees, your hands resting behind your neck (not intertwined) and the soles of your feet resting on the ground. Lift your head and shoulders 5-10 cm so that the shoulder blades are off the ground.
- Return without touching the floor, but always keeping half a centimeter off the ground, to keep the part constantly in tension.

- You could start by doing 3 sets of 10, week after week, to 3 sets of 15, up to 3 sets of 20: this is the recommended progression.
- Between one series and the next, I recommend a minute of rest for beginners, and 30 or 40 seconds for the more trained.
- Basically, I feel a cramp that tells me when the muscles are at the right training stimulus and therefore need recovery. Because if I don't recover completely, I can't do as many as well.

The Plank

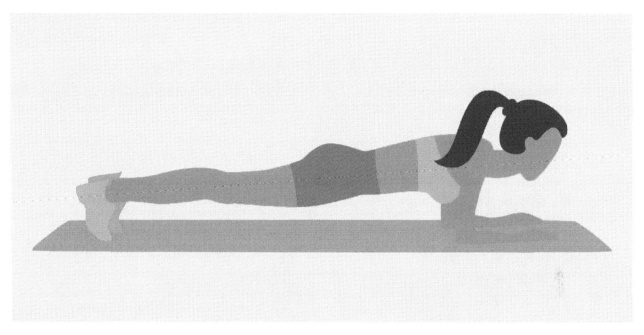

In the facilitated version, it can be done in the prone position with the arms outstretched resting on the hands below the height of the shoulders, the rest of the weight on the tips of the feet and the body completely stretched.

- The gaze is turned towards the line that joins the hands, with the position of the head neutral.
- Maintain the position for 20 seconds at the beginning, up to one minute as a progression of fatigue.
- Also, in this case it is necessary to evaluate one's own conditions. For example, a woman or an overweight man may feel all the fatigue on the arms and not on the abdomen: if you struggle too much, just hold the position for fewer seconds.
- Or again, you can lean on your knees, so as to decrease the weight on your arms.
- This is a complex exercise because it trains the deep muscle of the abdomen which is called the transverse: a sort of natural corset that gives stability to the back.

The Obliques

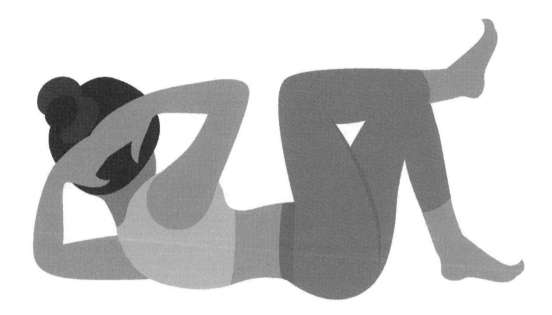

- Get in the same starting position as for the crunch,
- with the right leg crossed over the left knee,
- the left hand behind the neck and
- the right arm resting diagonally on the ground.
- Bring your left elbow in the direction of the bent right knee.
- The recommended repetition is 3 sets of 10 per side, with rest for one minute or 40 seconds.

Standing

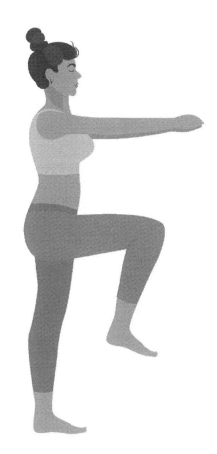

- The exercises for the abdomen can also be done standing, in order to facilitate the movement of bringing the knees to the chest.
- You have to put your right leg forward and left leg back with the heel raised, elbows at chest height with fingers intertwined.

- Keeping the elbows still, raise the left knee, as if to give a knee to the chest, and come back always keeping the opposite foot on the toe.
- Do 15 or 20 on each side, in this way work on the lower part of the abdomen.

Reverse Crunch

The reverse crunch is one of the most common and effective exercises for working out the abdominals. A simple exercise that will help tone and strengthen the whole core, the center of gravity of our body, responsible for all the actions of daily life such as walking, running, lifting and moving heavy objects.

Technically it is analogous to a normal crunch, with the difference that the torso will not go towards the legs, but the opposite, just as the name suggests, but we will talk about this shortly.

The muscle groups involved during reverse crunches are:

- Rectus abdominis
- Oblique
- Transverse abdominis
- Ileopsoas

The execution of this exercise will serve to strengthen these muscles in a profound way. Having a trained core is synonymous with balance and therefore with correct postural structure.

Correct execution and reverse crunch on the ground

To arrive at a correct execution of the reverse crunch it is essential to start from the right position.

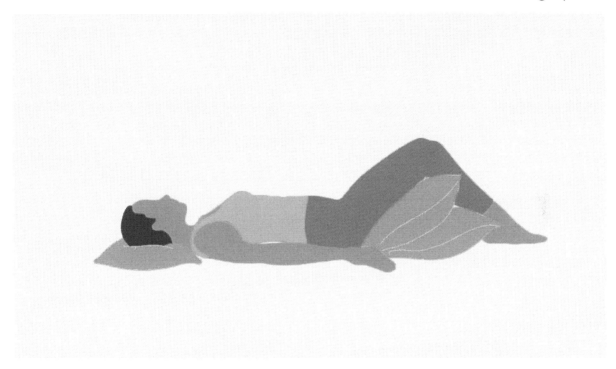

HERE'S HOW TO POSITION YOURSELF CORRECTLY:

- Lie on the floor or on a flat bench in supine position (on the back)
- The arms are extended at the sides with the palms resting on the ground
- The legs are parallel and slightly bent

INSTEAD, AS REGARDS THE CORRECT EXECUTION OF THE EXERCISE YOU MUST KEEP IN MIND THE FOLLOWING STEPS:

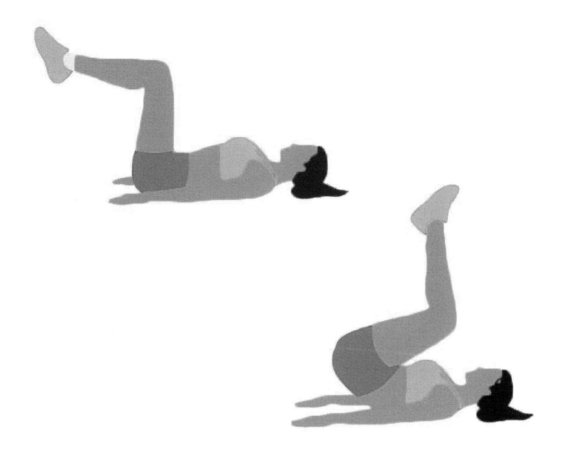

Raise both legs, keeping the knees flexed to form a 90° angle

The head and shoulders remain still, in a neutral position

With an abdominal contraction raise the pelvis, which curls up on itself and brings the knees towards the chest

Touching the point of maximum contraction, you return to the starting position: lowering the pelvis without arching the lumbar area and without losing contact with the floor.

APPLYING THE RIGHT BREATHING WHILE PERFORMING IS VERY IMPORTANT:

- Exhale during the abdominal contraction, when the pelvis rises so to speak
- Inhale during the descending phase of the legs.

Movement must be slow and controlled; do not perform the rebound to help the execution and do not completely bring the pelvis off the floor, keeping adherence only with the shoulder blades. If the first time you do the exercise it seems difficult, hold on to a fixed object and everything becomes easier.

The variations

Once you have learned the basic movement, you can intensify the exercise by integrating one of the following variations.

REVERSE CRUNCH ON A BENCH

It can be performed on a flat bench or an inclined bench. The method of execution remains the same.

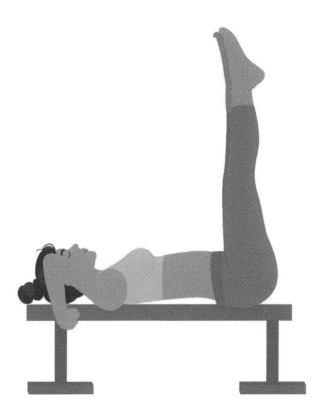

- Lie on a bench in the supine position
- Grab the edges of the bench at head level
- Raise your knees to 90 degrees
- Contract your core muscles and use your abs to lift your pelvis and knees towards your head

- Pause briefly in the high position of the movement and then slowly come down to the starting position
- A foam roller can also be placed in the crook of the knee by applying pressure while lifting the legs.

Exercises for Strengthening the Leg Muscles

EXERCISES FOR STRENGTHENING THE LEG MUSCLES ARE A FUNDAMENTAL ACTIVITY FOR THE ELDERLY.

It is one of the ways to keep balance in training and thus prevent the dangerous fall injuries to which we are all subject in old age. To facilitate the exercise of the elderly, you can opt for gentle gymnastic movements that can also be performed while sitting at home and without the support of special equipment.

Like any other type of training, even the ones dedicated to the elderly, they need consistency to achieve the desired effects.

Quadriceps and Knees

While sitting in a chair, keeping your back straight, lift one foot at a time, up to knee height. Repeat 5 times per leg.

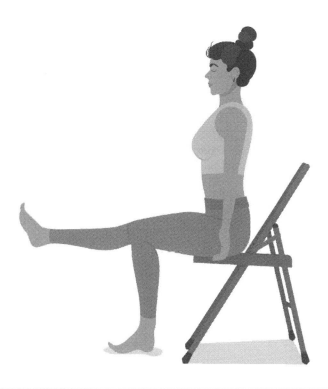

Calves

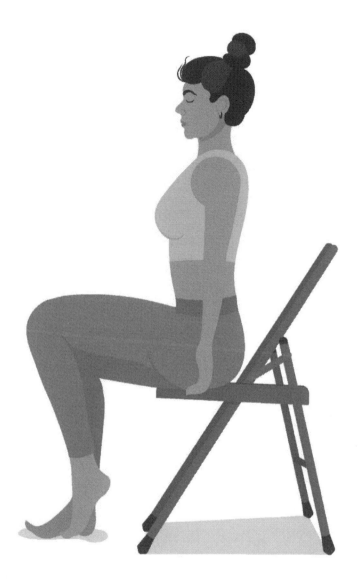

While sitting on a chair, lift your feet up on toes and lower them again, repeating the exercise 10 times per leg.

Calf Stretch

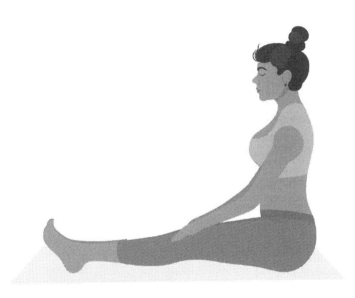

While sitting on the floor on a mat,
legs stretched forward, pull your toes
back and hold for 20 seconds.

Leg and Knee Stretch

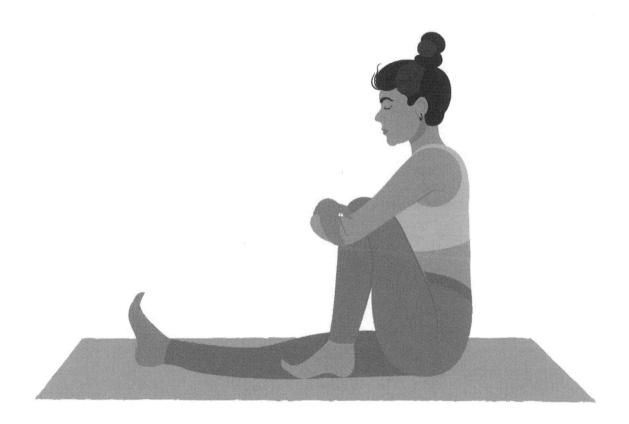

While sitting on the floor on a mat, legs extended forward, gently bring the knee of one leg to the chest, without excessive force. Maintain the position for 20 seconds per leg.

If practiced regularly, seated exercises for the leg muscles dedicated to the elderly, associated with an active life, bring benefits from the first weeks of practice.

Lateral Lift

CLASSICALLY USED FOR SHOULDER TRAINING, NOT MANY PEOPLE KNOW THE EFFECT OF THIS EXECUTION ON SYNERGISTIC AND DEEPER MUSCLES.

Moreover, a correct or incorrect technique - or simply a different one in the ROM or in the position of the arm - significantly changes the selectivity of muscle activation.

Let's see the details.

LATERAL RAISES: WHAT ARE THEY FOR?

The lateral lift is a monoarticular exercise (scapulo-humeral) aimed above all at the recruitment of the central or lateral deltoid muscle.

FUNCTION OF THE LATERAL DELTOID

The central deltoid abducts and flexes (especially with the arm internally rotated) up to 180°, it weakly participates in the extra rotation and horizontal extension of the arm.

LATERAL SHOULDER TRAINING IS MOSTLY AESTHETIC IN NATURE. Nevertheless, given the conspicuous activation of the supraspinatus, it also boasts discrete functional and preventive-rehabilitative applications.

THE TRAPEZIUS, large dentate (serratus anterior) and contralateral lumbar muscles should be less affected by movement, but not exempt. The use of the conditional mode will become clearer as the reading progresses.

Starting position of the side lift

The starting position is usually with an upright torso, head straight, with good lumbar support and activated shoulder blades.

When standing, the legs are naturally open or not wider than the shoulders; the knees must not be extended.

The arms naturally fall to the sides and the elbow is semi-flexed, meaning not extended but not bent.

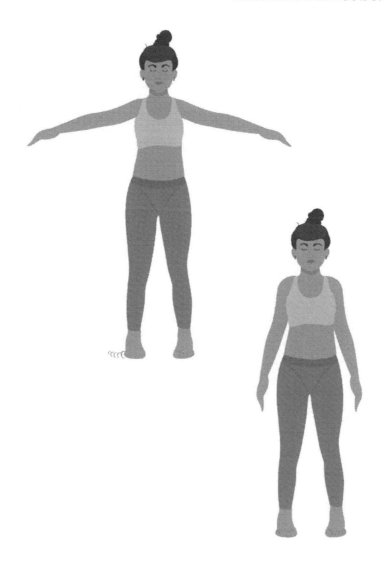

The lateral lift movement is an abduction in the frontal plane, starting at 0° (arms at the sides) and ending at 80-90°. The arm stops more or less parallel to the collarbones and we will better understand why below.

Note: the complete lift could continue up to 180°, as happens, for example, in the military press.

For a correct execution of the lateral lift, it is very important to consider the position of the humerus on its axis:

- If the lift is performed with the humerus positioned naturally, it is called neutral;
- If, on the other hand, the humerus rotates internally (with the thumb downwards) it is said to be in internal rotation;
- If, on the other hand, the humerus rotates externally it is called in external rotation.

But be careful, the fact that the humerus can be elevated in all three rotations does not mean that these movements have the same effect on the muscles and the joint.

LET'S START WITH THE FIRST CERTAINTY; the muscles are activated massively if the contraction starts from a condition of elongation. Conversely, if shortened, their stimulus is less intense. By turning inside, the central and especially the posterior deltoid start in a more elongated position.

However, it is indisputable that the physiological movement of abduction of the humerus involves extra rotation, especially beyond 80-90 By reducing the subacromial space, without extra-rotating, the head of the humerus no longer has room to move and, to prevent the movement from being interrupted, the movement of the scapula intervenes - up to that moment almost completely stationary.

Therefore, in the healthy subject with a normal-functional shoulder, the lateral lifts can be performed safely in a neutral or slightly intra-rotated position, up to an angle of 80-90°.

In compromised subjects, on the other hand, the best advice is to perform the lateral lift in a neutral or slightly external rotation position.

Variants of the side elevation

The side lift can be performed with free weights, then dumbbells or kettlebells, or even cables.

Moreover, the movement can involve the simultaneous use of both arms, that of one arm at a time, or even - rarely used - the alternating use of one limb and the other.

THE ONE-ARM SIDE LIFTS CAN ALSO BE DONE ON AN INCLINE BENCH, LYING ON YOUR SIDE.

Most common mistakes in side lifts

In the case of a painful shoulder, perhaps with a diagnosis of subacromial impingement syndrome, or even in the presence of limited excursion due to a particular joint morphology, performing the lateral lifts in internal rotation is undoubtedly a mistake.

NEGLECTING ANY PARA-PHYSIOLOGICAL OR PATHOLOGICAL CONDITIONS IS ALSO A MISTAKE. In case of hyperlordosis, for example, it is advisable to perform the lateral lift while seated rather than standing; even better if monolaterally. This is because, as we have anticipated, the lifting movement provides in itself a postural compensation for lumbar activation, to be avoided in those who show an evident excess of lordotic curvature.

ANOTHER CONSIDERABLE ERROR IS CONSTITUTED BY THE POSTURAL COMPENSATION (the classic lowering of the bust in the concentric phase), in the case inadequately high overloads are used.

Ground Crunch: Execution

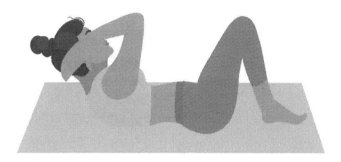

- **Lying on your back on the floor with knees bent so that both feet are resting on the floor with the entire sole. The lower limbs must remain motionless for the entire duration of the exercise.**
- **The head is initially in contact with the floor.**

- **Hands can be held at the sides, crossed across the chest, at the sides of the head at the temples, or behind the head with the shoulders fully flexed and the elbows extended.**

THE LIST WAS WRITTEN IN ASCENDING ORDER OF DIFFICULTY. Once established where to position the limbs, it is no longer possible to change this parameter except as a cheating technique or to lighten the load during a series in stripping.

The execution consists of performing a spine flexion so that the upper back comes off the floor, while the lower back remains in contact with the floor for the duration of the exercise.

The distance between the chin and the breastbone should remain as constant as possible.

The range of motion is reduced, as lifting the back too much ends up flexing the hip as well, turning the crunch into a sit-up. In case you are unable to keep your feet still on the floor, you need to switch to a lighter variant of crunch such as the one with hips flexed at 90° and feet resting on a raised surface. To emphasize the work of the oblique abdominals, it is possible to perform the concentric phase of the movement by twisting the torso towards the right side; in this movement the work of the external obliques of the left side and the internal obliques of the right side is maximized. The movement is one-sided and the description refers to the right side. Repeat in a mirror image for the left side.

The Russian twist

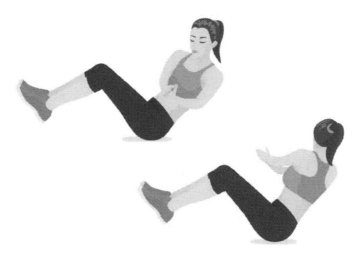

The Russian twist is an exercise that involves all the abdominal muscles, particularly effective for the waistline and to minimize the much-hated love handles: here is everything you need to know.

The Russian Twist is an exercise that allows you to fully activate the abdominals. This exercise trains the rectus abdominis, the obliques and the transversus abdomen, a muscle capable of stabilizing the spine and flattening the belly.

BENEFITS OF RUSSIAN TWIST

The Russian Twist strengthens the core, tones the central part of the body, slims the waist and reduces love handles. Ideal for improving balance, posture and torsion speed of the trunk. It does not require special tools, it's easy to learn and suitable for everyone thanks to the different execution variants.

WHAT IT TAKES TO PERFORM THE RUSSIAN TWIST

The Russian Twist can be performed on the ground using a mat or while sitting on a shelf or kneeling. To make the exercise more intense, you can hold dumbbells, kettlebells, balls, discs, medicine balls, water bottles, rubber bands in your hands.

With the Russian Twist exercise, you can also train the shoulders and arms, just add movements with the arms up, front diagonally, etc. to the torsion of the trunk, free body or with the use of external loads.

TIPS TO PERFORM THE RUSSIAN TWIST WITHOUT ERRORS

- Breathe deeply and steadily
- Exhale with each twist and inhale to return to center
- Engage your abdominal and back muscles
- Keep the body straight at a 45-degree angle from the floor and avoid bending and rolling
- Follow the movement of your hands with your eyes
- As you turn, bring your arms down as if to touch the floor next to you
- Use your abs to rotate left and right
- Create a V with the torso and thighs
- When you lift your feet, keep your balance on the buttocks and activate your core

Russian twist execution with feet resting

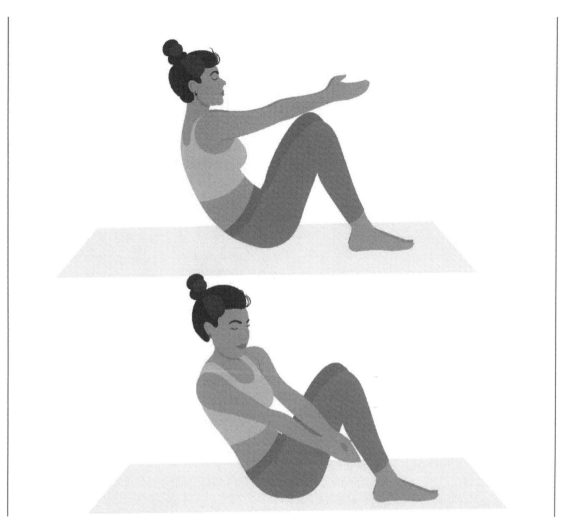

- Sit on the ground and keep your knees bent.
- Stretch and straighten your spine by creating a 45-degree angle from the floor.
- Bring your arms forward towards your chest, keep your elbows slightly bent and join your hands.
- Activate the abs and rotate the trunk to the right, return to the center and then rotate to the left.
- Do 2 to 3 sets of 10 to 20 repetitions. If you want to intensify the exercise, hold a load in your hands and hold it at chest height. Stretch the load down towards the floor or keep it at chest height while twisting.

Russian Twist execution with feet raised

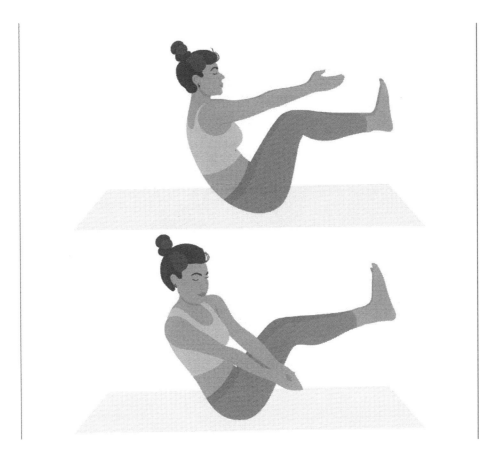

- Sit on the ground, keep your knees bent and lift your feet off the floor.
- Stretch and straighten your spine by creating a 45-degree angle from the floor.
- Bring your arms forward towards your chest, keep your elbows bent and join your hands.

- Activate the abs and rotate the trunk to the right, return to the center and then rotate to the left.
- Do 2 to 3 sets of 10 to 20 repetitions. If you want to intensify the exercise, hold a load in your hands and twist left and right, stretch the load down towards the floor or keep it at chest height while twisting.

Russian Twist execution with single leg extension

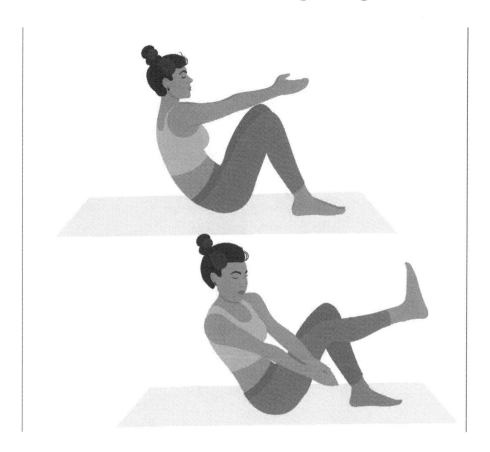

- Sit on the ground, keep your knees bent and lift your feet off the floor.
- Stretch and straighten your spine by creating a 45-degree angle from the floor.
- Bring your arms forward, keep your elbows bent and join your hands.
- Activate the abs, rotate the trunk to the right and straighten the right leg, return to the center and then rotate the trunk to the left and straighten the left leg.
- Do 2 to 3 sets of 10 to 20 repetitions. If you want to intensify the exercise, hold a load in your hands. Stretch the load down to the side towards the floor or keep it at chest height while twisting.

Performing Russian Twist Punch Blows

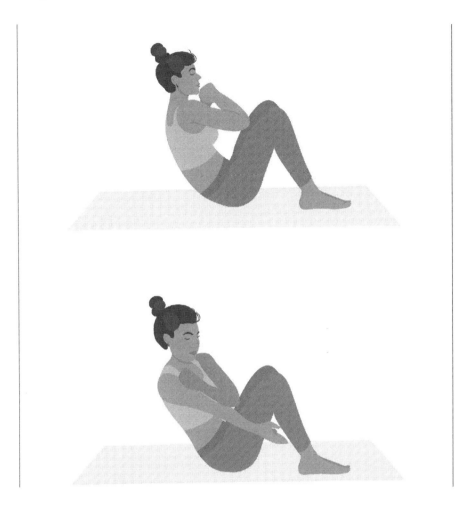

- Sit on the ground, keep your knees bent, you can do this exercise both with your feet on the ground and off the floor.
- Stretch and straighten your spine by creating a 45-degree angle from the floor.
- Keeping your arms folded in front of your chest activates your abs.

- Exhale, push and extends the left arm and twists with the trunk on the same side.
- Inhale and return to center.
- Exhale and repeat on the left side.
- Do 2 to 3 sets of 10 to 20 repetitions. If you want to intensify the exercise, hold some dumbbells in your hands.

Performing the Russian Twist with the movement of the arms

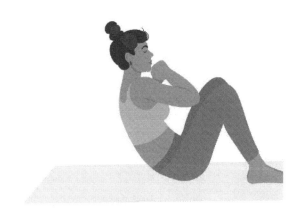

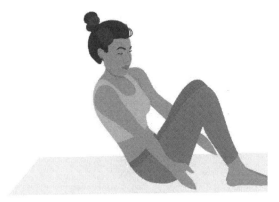

- Sit on the ground, keep your knees bent, you can do this exercise both with your feet on the ground and off the floor.
- Stretch and straighten your spine by creating a 45-degree angle from the floor.
- Keeping your arms folded in front of your chest activates your abs.
- Exhale, push and stretch your arms out to the side towards the floor as you twist with the trunk.
- Inhale as you return to the center position, as you raise your arms up towards the ceiling or extend them forward.
- Exhale and repeat the twist to the left.
- Do 2 to 3 sets of 10 to 20 repetitions. If you want to intensify the exercise, hold a load in your hands or place an elastic band on your wrists.

Russian Twist on a chair or bench

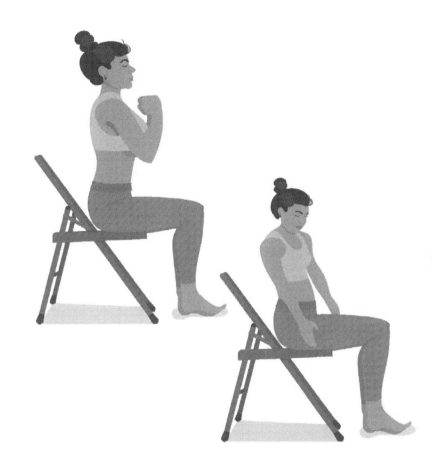

- Sit on a chair or bench and be sure to rest the soles of your feet on the floor.
- Bend your arms, join your hands and place them at chest height.
- Exhale, rotate the trunk to the right and stretch your arms towards the floor.

- Inhale, return to the starting position, and repeat to the left.
- Do 2 to 3 sets of 10 to 20 repetitions. If you want to intensify the exercise, hold a load in your hands or place an elastic band on your wrists.

Russian Twist on your knees

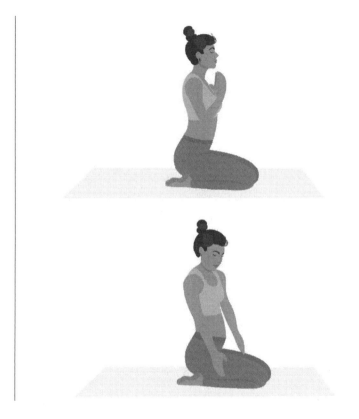

- Kneel on a mat or pillow.
- Bend your arms, join your hands and place them at chest height.
- Exhale, rotate the trunk to the right and stretch your arms towards the floor.
- Inhale return to the starting position and repeat to the left.
- Do 2 to 3 sets of 10 to 20 repetitions. If you want to intensify the exercise, hold a load in your hands or place an elastic band on your wrists.

HOW MANY TIMES A WEEK SHOULD THE RUSSIAN TWIST BE PERFORMED?

You can include this exercise in your daily workout routine. Do at least 3 sets. Choose the variant that suits your level. If you don't have enough balance and core stability, perform the Russian Twist initially without a load or with your feet resting on the floor.

If you want less strain on your back and hip flexors, start by doing the Russian Twist sitting on a chair or kneeling, and then move on to the next variations.

Abdominal Vacuum

THIS IS A TECHNIQUE TO TRAIN AT HOME OR WHEREVER YOU WANT, TO TONE THE ABDOMINALS, AND IN PARTICULAR THE TRANSVERSUS MUSCLE, THAT DEEP MUSCULATURE THAT HOLDS THE ORGANS IN AND THAT FLATTENS THE BELLY, ALLOWING A CORRECT POSTURE.

Less demanding than a tiring crunch or burpees session, it should not be underestimated. It is necessary to learn the correct execution technique and to be able to perform it well, which is essential in order to obtain good results.

Practiced consistently every day, it promises visible results after just a few weeks!

THE BENEFITS OF THE ABDOMINAL VACUUM

Even before being strictly physical exercise, it is self-awareness work that does not stress the body.

Everyone can do it: women and men of any age and even those with back or neck problems. Indeed, in these subjects, by improving posture and core tone, they will benefit.

THE IMPORTANT THING IS TO BE ABLE TO COORDINATE MUSCLE CONTRACTION AND BREATHING. Promises a toned flat stomach. And it is true, but in reality, the benefits it brings are much more. Let's see in more detail:

- It does not stress either the spinal column or the cervical ones
- It has no impact on the back
- It helps relieve stress
- It improves posture
- It oxygenates body and brain
- It calms the vegetative nervous system (the body's automatic functions such as digestion, respiration, circulation, etc ...)
- It reduces abdominal diastasis
- It improves body stability
- It increases the strength of the abdominal belt
- It stimulates the perineum
- It flattens the belly
- It stimulates abdominal peristalsis
- It is convenient because it can be performed in any place and at any time

MUSCLES INVOLVED IN THE VACUUM: Using breathing and contraction, this exercise activates and strengthens the abdominal-transverse muscle, the deepest part of the abdominal muscle. The transverse is of fundamental importance as it brings the viscera inwards and allows you to have correct posture and stability, the so-called core stability, or the stability of the trunk.

Apparently simple, to do it in the right way, you need to do a lot of practice. HERE ARE THE INDICATIONS FOR THE CORRECT EXECUTION:

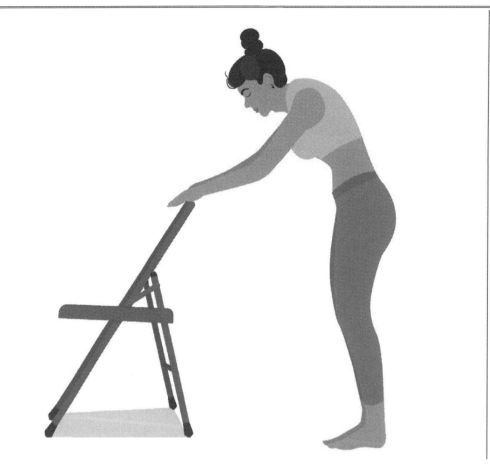

- Stand up, legs slightly bent and shoulder width apart
- Place your hands on a table or a support surface that is level with the pelvis (or simply leave your arms at your sides)
- Bend the torso a little forward
- Inhale deeply until your lungs are filled with air

- Push out all the air by making it come out first from the belly and then from the lungs
- Pull the abdomen in while exhaling, as if wanting to bring the navel closer to the spine
- Hold this position for at least 5 seconds without inhaling
- Relax and breathe normally for 1 or 2 minutes, then inhale and repeat the exercise

The benefits of this technique can be amazing!

How many times?

The ideal is to perform the exercise every day for 5-15 times in a row. At first, hold the position for 5 seconds and then gradually increase up to 30 seconds by taking small breaths.

Abdominal vacuum lying down

Let's now see the simplest technique and therefore recommended for beginners.

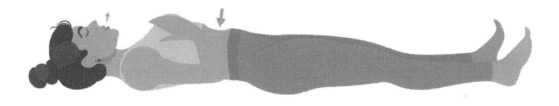

Here's how to do it: lie on the ground on your back, hands resting on the stomach, inhale by inflating the belly and exhale by sucking the navel towards the spine.

Variant in quadrupedal

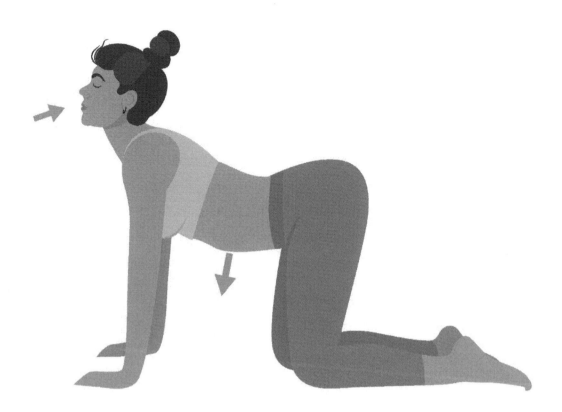

Assume the quadrupedal position (on all fours), inhale by releasing the belly towards the floor and exhale by **pushing the belly in while keeping the lower back firmly.**

MORE DIFFICULT VARIANTS

After the first initial stages, which are essential for becoming familiar with the exercise and understanding how to breathe and how to 'move' the belly, it is possible to move on to more difficult variants that make the exercise more intense.

The exercise is always the same, but the positions in which it is performed vary, no longer from the supine position but:

- In quadrupedal
- Sitting on a chair
- On a fit ball
- Standing with the torso bent forward

HOW LONG DOES IT TAKE TO SEE RESULTS WITH THE ABDOMINAL VACUUM?

If done consistently and correctly, it brings visible and satisfying results within 3 weeks.

It is not an exercise that replaces the classic crunches, and the plank, but a complementary one that should be present in any training program.

TIPS AND WARNINGS FOR THE ABDOMINAL VACUUM

It is preferable to do it in the morning on an empty stomach, or in any case between meals (you risk regurgitation).

Not recommended in case of inguinal hernia.

Start gradually and slowly increase the hold as you train.

The first few times perform the simpler variations: lying down or on all fours.

For a truly optimal result, in terms of a flat stomach, it must be combined with a healthy, balanced and controlled diet.

Once you understand the execution technique well, perform the exercise several times throughout the day, even while sitting or standing.

MISTAKES TO AVOID IN THE ABDOMINAL VACUUM

At the beginning, avoid keeping the abdomen contracted for more than 5 seconds, and catch your breath well before doing another repetition.

Be careful not to run out of oxygen, the risk could be that of sudden dizziness.

Exercises to Strengthen the Hips

1 - Front split

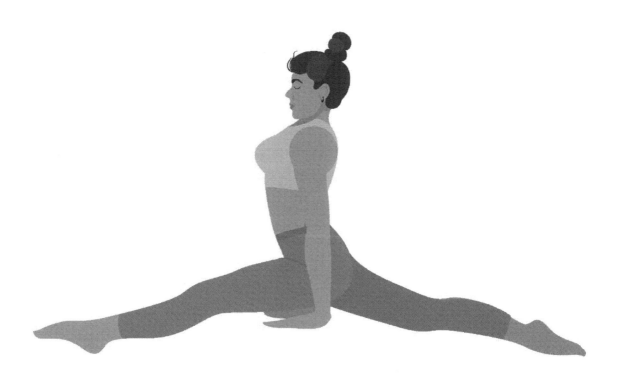

Open your legs by spreading them, placing your hands on the ground to maintain balance and correct posture of the back. Do not force excessively but keep the static working position with slight tension on the inner thigh. The feet should be parallel and the knees kept straight.

2 – Sun

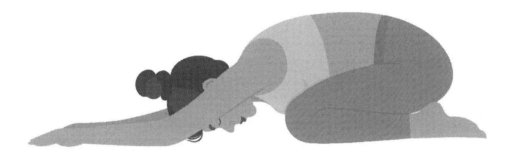

From the previous position, with the help of your hands, place your knees on the ground in a position of maximum spread between them. Close the feet by bending the knees and bringing the soles of the feet in contact with each other. By placing the elbows on the ground, keep the back straight with the core and actively push the pelvis downwards, increasing the opening of the hip.

3 - Frog bust erect

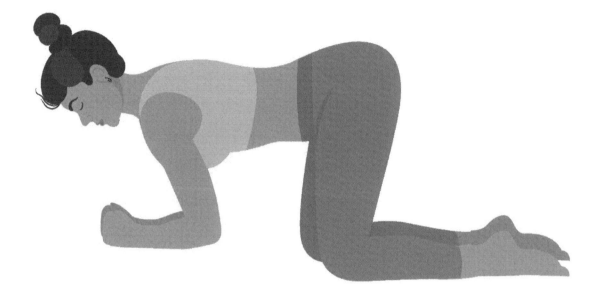

From the previous position, rotate the hips, bringing the torso straight without changing the position of the legs and feet. Maintain the correct position of the torso.

4 - Lateral Sphinx

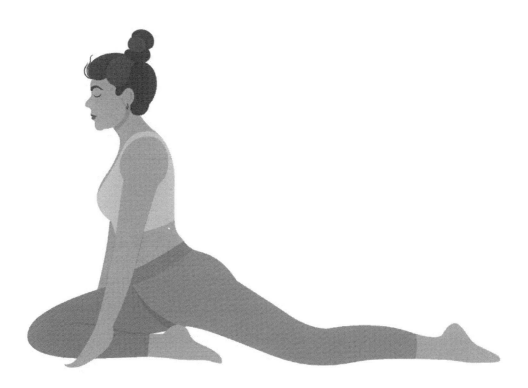

Extend one leg sideways bringing the straight leg with the cut foot. Open the thigh of the flexed knee bringing the angle between the legs to the maximum of your opening. Keep the trunk as erect as possible.

5 - Lateral sphinx with hammer foot

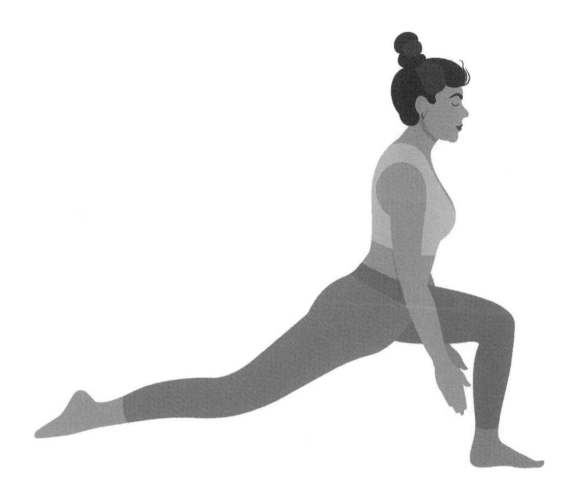

Keeping the position of the leg and trunk still, rotate the straight leg bringing the hammer foot with the toe upwards. Be careful not to sit back.

6 - Lateral sphinx rotations straight leg

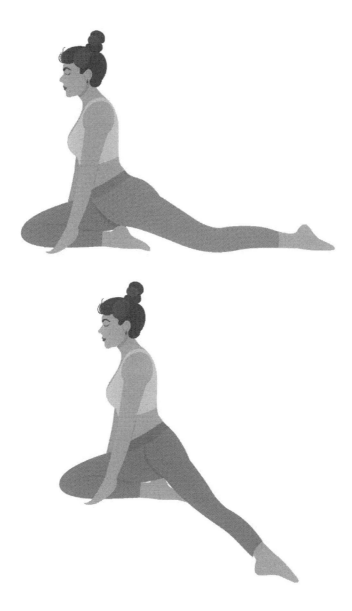

Keeping the bent leg still, make 180° rotations of the straight leg. From foot to hammer position to back of foot on the ground. Rotate your hips from front to side. Be careful not to tilt your torso and isolate it from the rest.

Repeat routine 4 to 6 with the other limb.

7 - Frontal split with hammer feet

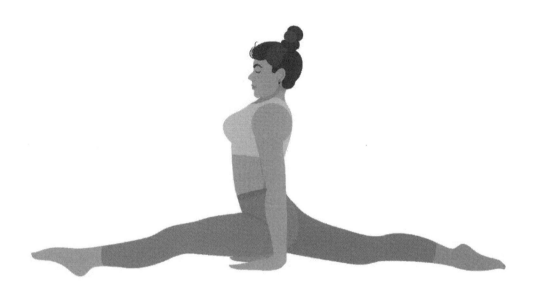

By widening the bent leg from the position under the pelvis, find the maximum frontal spread resting on the heels and the toes upwards. I recommend using the support of the hands to avoid dangerous balance losses in maximum spread.

8 - Sagittal splits

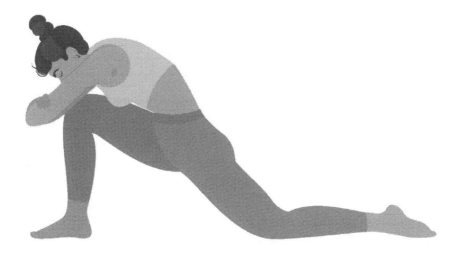

From the front split position, rotate the hip and lean sideways on the heel of the front leg and on the back of the foot and the knee of the rear leg. Possibly keep the trunk erect. Repeat the operation on the opposite side, using your arms to change the position.

9 - Front sitting split

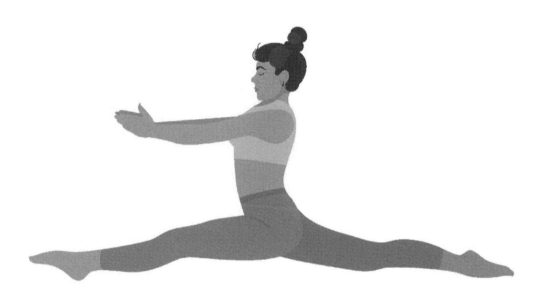

Returning to the front spread position, using your hands to sit backwards without losing the opening of the legs in the sitting spread position. Keep your torso erect.

10 - Seated front split with straight arms

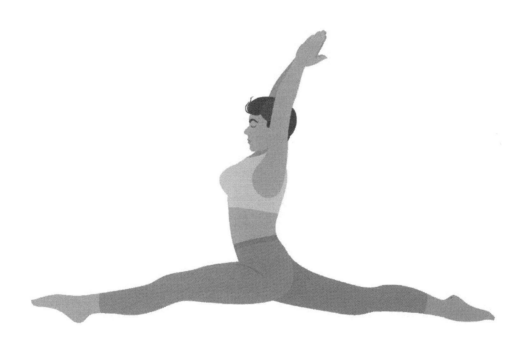

Remaining in the spread position on the ground, bring your arms upward while keeping your torso erect.

11 - Front splits, lateral torso flexion

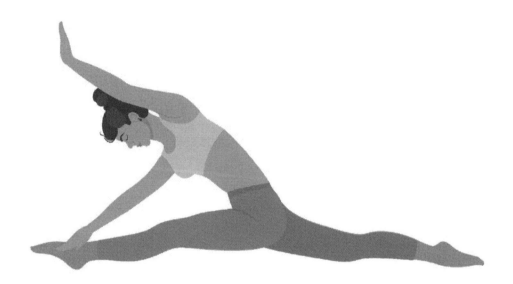

Keeping the legs locked to the ground with the hammer feet, bring the torso sideways with the front arm (from the flexion side) in front of the abdomen and the opposite hand from above the head towards the crossed foot. Repeat the operation on the opposite side.

12 - Frontal splits bending of the front torso

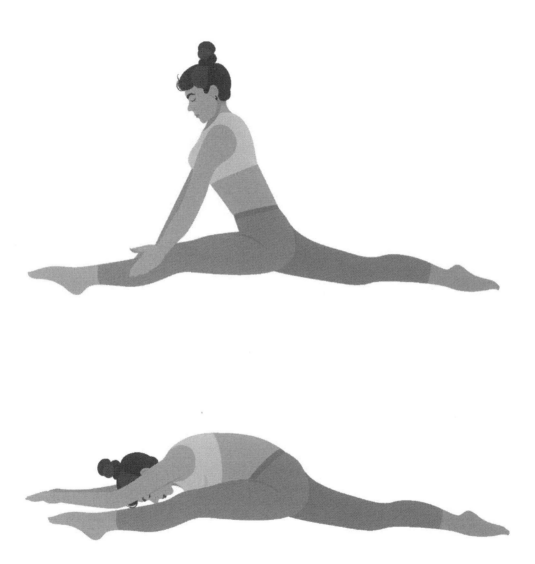

Bring both arms forward towards the ground, with the idea of reaching for something far in front of us. The bust is very straight, working on the mobility of the hip and not on the flexion of the curved back.

13 - Sole pelvis forward

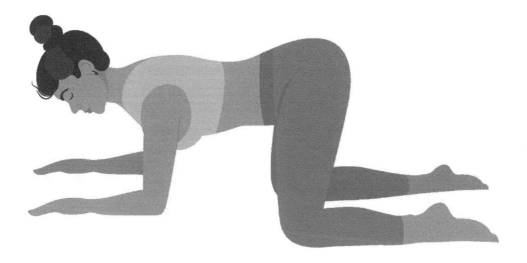

From the previous position, with the help of your hands, lean back in a spread and then, placing your knees on the ground, return to the sole position and then bring the pelvis forward by springing back and forth on the axis of the torso. The idea is to bring the pelvis closer and further away from the feet without changing the distance of the same from the ground.

14 – Frog

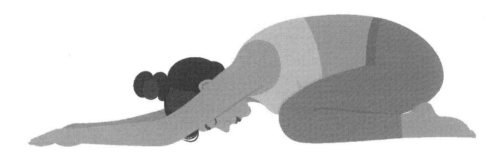

Opening the angle of the legs, bending the knees imitating the Shiko dachi position. Maintain the position by actively pushing the pelvis towards the ground.

15 - 1/2 open leg frog

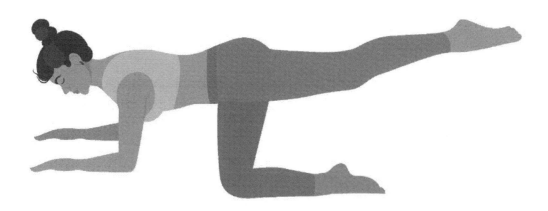

From the previous position, alternately bring the leg with the foot upwards, approaching the pelvis from that side to the ground.

METHODS OF EXECUTION:

It is recommended to maintain the static stretch position for at least 30/40 mins.

Depending on the reason for which we train, we can repeat the exercises for several series.

If I want to significantly improve joint mobility, at least 3 series are essential if, on the other hand, I simply want to stretch the muscles concerned without particular development, one series will be more than enough.

Have a good workout and open your hips!

How to Do Diaphragmatic Breathing

When you train for strength, adequate breathing is essential to achieve the desired results. By following the right techniques, you will guarantee your muscles the oxygen they need, thus increasing your performance. Here's how to breathe properly during sports and what mistakes to avoid.

The basic principles of breathing

Without nourishment, water and rest, we could only survive for a certain amount of time. But what living beings really can't do without is breathing, the most natural act in the world: practically no one stops to reflect on their own breathing. Almost without realizing it, through the nose or mouth we introduce air into our lungs up to about 200,000 times a day, and then expel it again.

Through inhalation, our body takes in oxygen, an essential element for all metabolic processes, which is transported to the organs and cells through the circulatory system.

On exhaling, the air that has reached the lungs is expelled through the mouth and nose. Specifically, in addition to carbon dioxide, other waste of metabolic processes, such as nitrogen, are also expelled.

The muscles involved in inhalation and exhalation are numerous. The diaphragm, the muscle located below the lungs, which separates the thoracic cavity from the abdominal cavity, plays the main role. By contracting, the diaphragm ensures that the chest rises or falls or, as occurs in the so-called abdominal breathing, that the abdomen arches forward and then contract inwards.

The importance of breathing in muscle training

Those who remain seated for a long time in a room where the air is stale will feel increasingly tired and lose concentration over time. In most cases it is sufficient to ventilate the room briefly to regain new energy. The principle is also similar for the muscles: in order to carry out their activity without getting tired ahead of time, our muscles cannot do without oxygen. The greater the effort we put on our body, the greater the amount of oxygen needed by our muscle tissues.

But that's not all, because following the right breathing technique during strength training can increase performance. In fact, correct breathing will help you keep the torso (or core) contracted and ensure the right stability: a decisive factor, especially when you train with heavy weights. The more stable your body is, the more strength you will be able to generate, thus improving your performance. Each repetition will be more effective and progress will not be long in coming.

Conversely, improper breathing could lead to problems and injuries. In case of shallow breathing, the muscle tension will be less and, consequently, your cells will not receive enough oxygen. Holding the air too long could then compromise pulmonary veins and alveoli due to excessive tension. In the worst case, severe oxygen deficiency could even result in fainting.

Strength training: the right breathing

Any physical activity, from running to weight lifting, causes an increase in breathing rate. Your breaths will become closer and more intense as, due to the strain your body is subjected to, you will need more oxygen.

PROPER BREATHING DURING STRENGTH TRAINING IS BASED ON THREE PRINCIPLES.

THE KEY RULE IS SIMPLE: exhale during the concentric phase (i.e. muscle contraction) and inhale during the eccentric phase (release and relaxation). Let's take a practical example: practicing the bench press you will have to exhale as you lift the weight and inhale as you bring it back down.

EVEN IN TIMES OF GREATEST EXERTION, TRY TO KEEP TAKING SLOW, DEEP BREATHS. Breathing intensely even at lower frequencies, for example during the rest phases, will only bring you benefits: by doing so you will constantly train the muscles involved in breathing and you can then apply the same technique even when you train.

Also learn to perform abdominal breathing, which requires much less effort than normal breathing, which occurs in the chest and shoulders. With this technique you will simultaneously inhale more oxygen with each breath; it will also allow you to lower blood pressure and aid digestion.

FREEDIVING: BENEFITS AND RISKS

Many athletes are convinced that holding their breath during strength training can bring benefits: in the moment of greatest effort, between inhalation and exhalation, they practice a moment of voluntary apnea. This strategy has its advantages, but it also carries several risks.

THE ADVANTAGES OF FREEDIVING

By retaining the air, the core muscles contract and, during the effort, the body acquires greater stability. Your muscles will also have access to new oxygen to coincide with the peak of their performance. Conversely, when inhaling and exhaling the muscle tissue cells are weaker.

THE RISKS OF APNEA

Apnea, however, causes an increase in pressure on the heart, which is why it should be avoided in people suffering from high blood pressure or cardiovascular disease.

If the breath is held for too long, this practice can give rise to cardiovascular problems even in healthy athletes. And here another risk could arise: the expulsion of waste elements, such as carbon dioxide and lactic acid, is temporarily blocked and your muscles could reach excessive levels of acidity. The consequence? Muscle aches and cramps.

Furthermore, you should never inhale or exhale at the peak of the effort (for example, when you reach the lowest point of the squat) or the strength in the muscles may be reduced.

Breathing is a fundamental element of strength training: it guarantees the muscles an adequate supply of oxygen and allows you to increase performance.

The right breathing technique ensures stability at the level of the torso, and also helps athletes to get the most out of individual repetitions.

THE KEY RULE IS ONE: EXHALE AT THE MOMENT OF CONTRACTION AND INHALE WHEN THE MUSCLES ARE RELEASED.

Abdominal breathing is particularly effective for giving greater stability to the core during training.

The diaphragm is the main muscle used in breathing and expands throughout the chest cavity. It is shaped like a slightly flattened double dome and is located just below the lungs and heart.

It lowers during inhalation, creating a vacuum effect that pushes the air into the lungs, while it returns to rest rising during exhalation, forcing the expulsion of carbon dioxide from the lungs.

THE BREATHING PROCESS: THE DIAPHRAGM LOWERS DURING INHALATION AND RISES DURING EXHALATION

The diaphragm does most of the work during the inhalation part, contracting so that the lungs can expand and take in all the necessary air. The muscles between the ribs, known as the intercostal muscles, lift the rib cage to help the diaphragm get enough air into the lungs.

Diaphragmatic breathing as just described is the natural and spontaneous state of breathing, but more and more people develop during their life a thoracic breathing, much less deep than the diaphragmatic one, not physiological and consequently limiting for the correct functioning of our organs.

WHY DO WE BREATHE FROM THE CHEST?

The cause of this impaired breathing (thoracic) is often the stressful lifestyle we are subjected to, which affects our breathing literally causing us to hold our breath and block the diaphragm in the lower part of the chest, never allowing air to flow freely and causing a natural retraction of the diaphragm which also affects the other muscles involved in the respiratory process.

To understand if you are using the diaphragm to its full potential, just place one hand on your stomach and one on your chest while you breathe: if you feel your belly expanding outwards when you are inhaling, while the chest remains relatively motionless, it means that you are breathing correctly with your diaphragm. If, on the other hand, it is the chest that expands while the belly remains almost still, your breathing is thoracic and must be corrected.

CONSEQUENCES OF IMPROPER BREATHING

By breathing with the chest and thus limiting the movement space of the diaphragm, you can face very serious consequences that involve muscles and organs that interact (directly or indirectly) with the diaphragm. Some of the problems related to chest breathing are:

- Breathing problems (for example asthma)
- Circulation problems
- Lower back pain
- Incorrect posture
- Digestive problems
- Accumulation of pain in the neck, shoulders and upper back
- Tension of the facial muscles

BENEFITS OF DIAPHRAGMATIC BREATHING

In addition to eliminating the harmful effects of chest breathing, diaphragmatic breathing brings with it numerous benefits. Being the basis of meditation, it exerts an indirect influence on all the benefits related to it, but even if practiced outside the meditative disciplines it has an incredible impact on body and mind. Here are some of its benefits:

- Helps you relax, reducing the harmful effects of cortisol (the stress hormone) on your body
- Slows down the heart rate, and is therefore very useful for those suffering from tachycardia
- Helps to lower blood pressure
- Helps you cope with the symptoms of post-traumatic stress disorder (PTSD)
- Improve muscle stability
- Improves resistance to intense physical exercise, and is therefore ideal for athletes
- Reduces the risk of muscle injuries and strains
- Slows down the rate of breathing and consequently helps to save energy

Exercises to train diaphragmatic breathing

Like any other muscle in the body, the diaphragm also needs to be trained in order to work to its full potential. If you are not belly breathing, here are a series of exercises you can perform to loosen, stretch and strengthen the diaphragm, radically changing the way you breathe:

Diaphragmatic breathing position

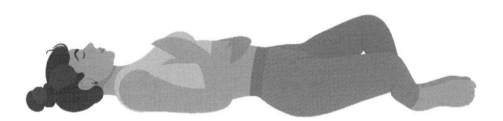

- Lie on the floor on your back - you can use a yoga mat or blanket if necessary for added comfort, but make sure the surface you rest on is not overly soft.
- Bend your legs and place your feet about 20 centimeters apart, with the soles firmly resting on the ground.

- Relaxing the whole body, place one hand on the stomach and the other on the chest.
- Start breathing through your nose, trying to raise only the hand resting on your stomach with each inhalation.
- Exhale through your mouth, continuing to focus on the movements of your body.
- Repeat for ten breaths.

Strengthen the diaphragm

Exercise to strengthen the diaphragm with hands on the sides of the rib cage

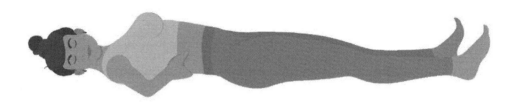

- Lie down supine on the floor (you can help yourself with a blanket or a support mat).
- Place both hands around the base of the rib cage, with the thumbs resting on the sides of the chest, facing the floor (they should touch the last rib on the side of the chest) and the other fingers extended along the chest. If you have a small rib cage the fingers of both hands may also touch.
- Press your thumbs against the ribs to get a slight resistance to their movement.
- Concentrate on expanding the rib cage as much as you can, so that the ribs press against the thumbs.

- Keep your eyes open initially so you can see the movement of the diaphragm as it expands.
- With each inhalation, slightly move your hands away from each other and bring them closer together when you exhale.
- Continue to breathe in this way, resisting the expansion of the rib cage, for ten breaths.
- Once the cycle is complete, extend your arms to the ground at your sides and breathe another ten times.
- Repeat the exercise for two more cycles.
- Try to generate a harmonious and uniform movement, not a mechanical one.

SANDBAG BREATHING

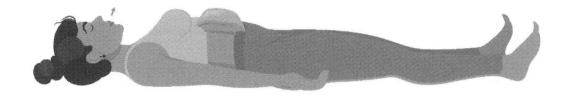

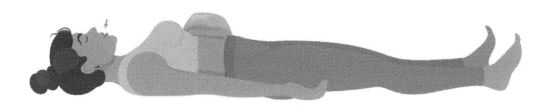

For this exercise you will need a bag of sand (or similar materials, such as beans or seeds) weighing about 4 pounds.

Lie on the floor on your back.

Place the sandbag at the base of your rib cage, under your pecs. The sac should cover the area that goes from the middle of the ribs to the abdomen, just above the navel.

Begin directing your breathing to the area where the sac is located, with the purpose of raising and lowering it as you inhale and exhale.

Try not to lift the body by force with the muscles, but gradually expand it through inhalation to the point of lifting the bag.

Continue lifting the bag through the breath for ten breaths, then rest for another ten breaths.

Repeat for two more sets.

Conclusion

Breathing stimulates the whole body to work better, which is why it has such a profound effect on our general well-being.

The diaphragm is an organ that plays a fundamental role in the breathing process and, when it is free from constrictions and alterations, it can generate an expansion that massages, stimulates and supplies all the surrounding organs and tissues with blood and oxygen.

Benefits of stretching

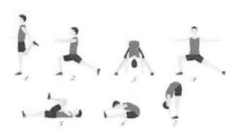

Stretching is essential not only when training, to lengthen the muscles and more: here are all the benefits and exercises recommended for a gentle but effective stretch

Stretching is an exercise technique that lengthens and improves muscle elasticity, lubricates joints, corrects posture, oxygenates cells, reactivates blood circulation, eliminates waste, prevents trauma, reduces inflammation and pain, brings the body towards complete physical well-being.

When a muscle shortens and loses its flexibility, it creates greater wear on the articular cartilage: with the practice of stretching, it is possible to reduce muscle tension, regenerate joints, tendons and bones.

A contracted muscle, in fact, by compensation, stresses and compromises the other parts of the body. This situation can lead to lower performance during training and an increased risk of injury. Practicing stretching before and after training increases the range of movement of the body during actions that are carried out in the workplace or in everyday life, improves fitness and athletic performance, and not least, leads to greater physical and mental awareness.

Let's see in detail all its benefits.

Effects and benefits of stretching on the body

Eliminates toxins and improves the appearance of the skin and capillaries

A muscle that stretches regularly helps improve blood and lymphatic circulation in that particular area of the body. With the increase in circulatory flow, the disposal of lactic acid and waste that accumulate in the blood and cells is favored: this leads to a reduction in water retention, smoother skin and less fragile capillaries.

It fights joint stiffness that often causes pain

Stretching exercises make muscles, tendons and joints more flexible. The flexibility and better lubrication helps prevent and improve various degenerative situations such as osteoarthritis and cartilage wear, and also osteoporosis.

Improve physical potential

With stretching exercises, it is possible to understand and improve one's motor and joint limits: thanks to stretching it is possible to reduce trauma and enhance strength, speed and endurance.

Brings physical and mental well-being

Muscle stretching improves the entire flexibility of the body and mind because good elasticity leads to improving the quality of daily movements and allows you to do things more easily, without the fear of getting stuck.

Dynamic and static stretching: the techniques

The best-known stretching techniques are classified into two types: dynamic and static. Let's see them in detail.

DYNAMIC STRETCHING (PRE-WORKOUT)

Dynamic stretching is often done as a form of warm-up because it helps raise the body's temperature and increases blood flow. Dynamic stretches prepare the muscles and joints to extend gradually and to cope with training without stress.

The movements in dynamic stretching are performed in an active and controlled way. The exercises slowly bring the muscles and joints to reach their natural width and length, through:

- oscillations,
- rotational movements,
- extensions,
- push-ups and
- hops.

You can choose to perform a dynamic stretch only in the part of the body you need to train. In the initial phase, perform the exercises slowly and gradually increase the speed of the movement.

Example of dynamic stretching for the shoulders

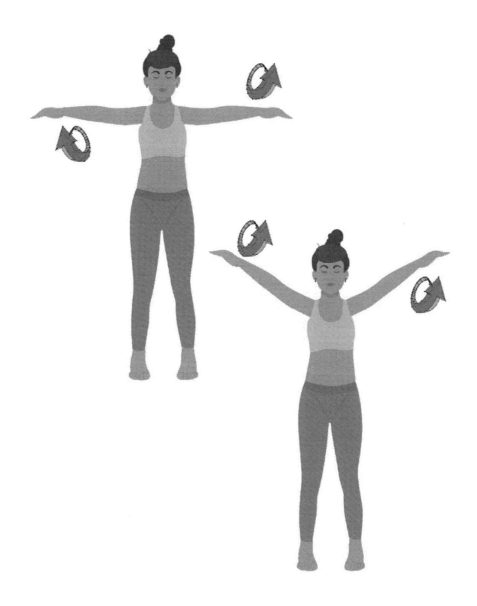

In an upright position, open and extend your arms to the sides until you feel the shoulder joint moving towards a natural and gradual opening. Make circulatory movements clockwise for 1 minute and counterclockwise for another 1 minute.

STATIC STRETCHING (POST-WORKOUT)

Static stretching leads to stretching the body in a progressive way until reaching the maximum stretching of the muscles, tendons and joints. It should be practiced with a medium-high body temperature, so it should be done after training.

Static stretching improves joint mobility and range of motion, leads the body to move without difficulty in everyday life, allows you to increase physical performance and the ability to perform exercises correctly, without straining too much muscles and joints. in addition, it helps to dispose of lactic acid.

Attention: Stretching must be achieved without achieving the sensation of pain. While reaching the stretch, you need to breathe calmly.

BREATHING DURING STATIC STRETCHING

During the stretch phase, which should last about 5-8 seconds, you exhale. When you reach the maximum stretch point you inhale and then continue to breathe naturally. It remains in the stretch point for 20-30 seconds up to a maximum of 1 minute.

TIPS FOR A GOOD STRETCH

- Stay focused
- Wear comfortable clothing and a suitable mat
- Avoid comparing your performance to that of others
- Do not bounce while assuming positions
- Always do a general warm-up phase before starting static stretching
- Maintain constant stretching for a time ranging from 20 to 60 seconds
- Stretch out by feeling your breath and your body's maximum degree of stretch
- Improve your flexibility gradually and without jerks
- Be consistent: Do at least 10 minutes of stretching at the end of each workout
- Don't think of stretching as a boring and useless thing!

Neck pain? Here is effective stretching to help you relax and feel better

Stretching to improve neck flexibility

Relieving neck tension has benefits throughout the upper body, from the shoulders to the spine. Repeat each exercise 2 times.

Exercise 1

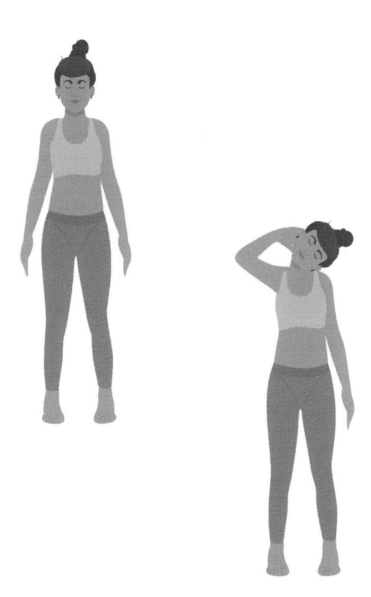

You can perform this position standing or sitting: let an ear fall towards the shoulder, apply light pressure with the hand on the head. Keep it there for 30 to 60 seconds. Repeat on the opposite side.

Exercise 2

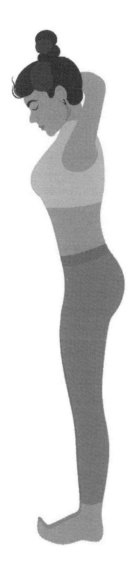

You can perform this position standing or sitting. Bring your hands behind your head and cross them. Apply light pressure and push your chin towards your chest. Remain in this position for 30 to 60 seconds.

Exercise 3

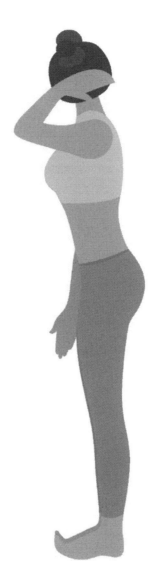

You can perform this position standing or sitting. Stand with your back firm and straight, place one hand behind your head and slowly turn your head to one side, apply light pressure and bring your chin towards your shoulder. Remain in position for 30 to 60 seconds. Repeat on the opposite side.

Exercise 4

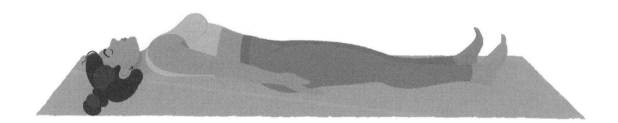

Lie on your back, bring your hands to your sides, lift your elbows and slowly raise your shoulders, bring your chest forward and slightly push your head back, rest the top of your head gently on the ground. Stay in position for 30 to 60 seconds.

Shoulder stretch

Stretching the shoulders improves poor posture and relieves tension in the shoulder blades, neck and upper body.

Exercise 5

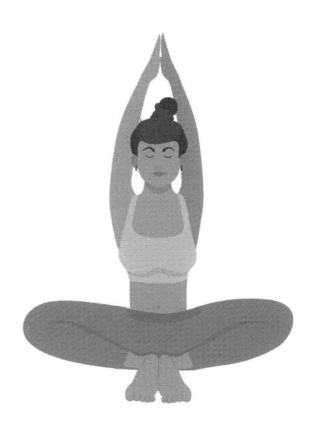

Sit comfortably, join your hands together, straighten and stretch your arms over your head. Squeeze your shoulder blades, remain for 10 seconds, rest a few seconds and repeat 5 times.

Exercise 6

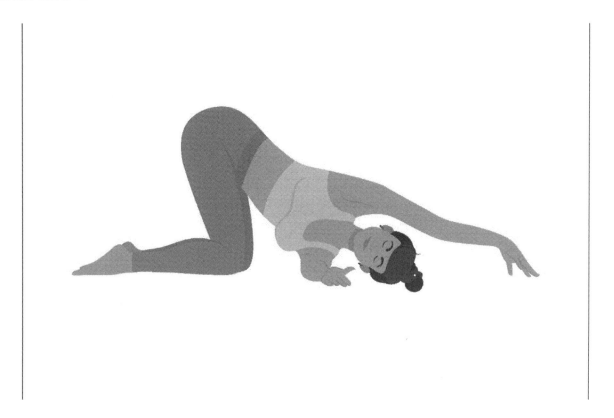

Get on all fours, with your buttocks high, rotate your trunk and gently slide your arm towards the floor until your shoulder and head rest on the ground. Apply light pressure on the arm to allow the shoulder to stretch. Remain in this position for 30 to 60 seconds. Repeat on the opposite side. Do the sequence 2 times.

Exercise 7

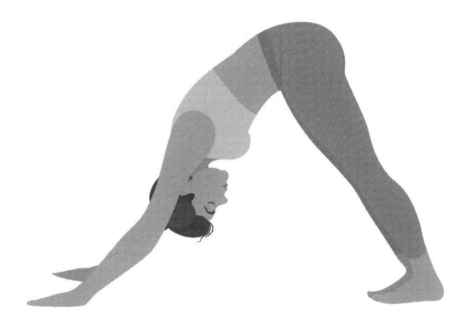

From the 4-legged position, lift your knees off the ground and push your glutes up. Stay with your glutes high, stretch your back and arms forward. Bring your heels to the floor and your head in your arms. Bring your shoulder blades together and feel the stretch in your shoulders. Hold for 30 seconds and repeat 2 times.

Exercise 8

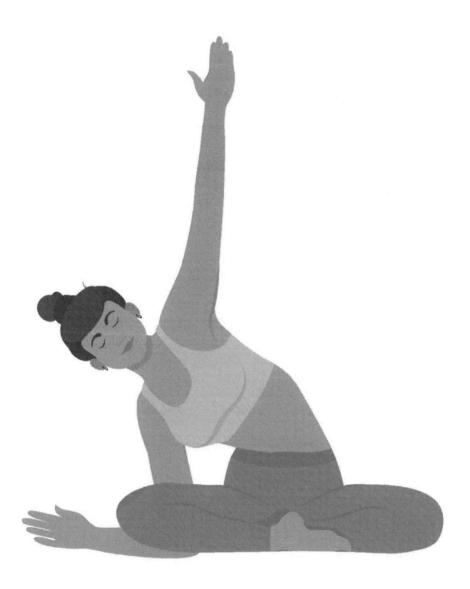

Sit down and lean to one side until your elbow and forearm rest on the ground. Stay with your glutes on the ground as you slowly extend your arm near your ear. Stay 30 to 60 seconds, and repeat on the other side. Do the exercise 2 times.

Leg stretch

Stretching the legs improves blood circulation and reduces the feeling of heavy and tired legs. Having more elasticity in the legs, it relieves tensions in the pelvis and prevents sciatica and piriformis syndrome.

Exercise 9

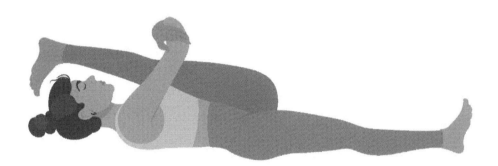

Lie on your back: hug one leg towards your chest and try to keep the rest of your body on the ground. Stay in position for 30 to 60 seconds. Repeat on the other leg. Do the sequence 2 times.

Exercise 10

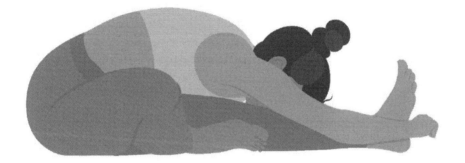

Forward bend

Sit comfortably, put the sole of one foot inside the inner thigh of the other leg and put it straight out in front of you. Slowly lean forward and come down as far as you can, grab a point on your foot or leg with your hands and stay for 30 to 60 seconds. Repeat on the other side. Do the sequence 2 times.

Exercise 11

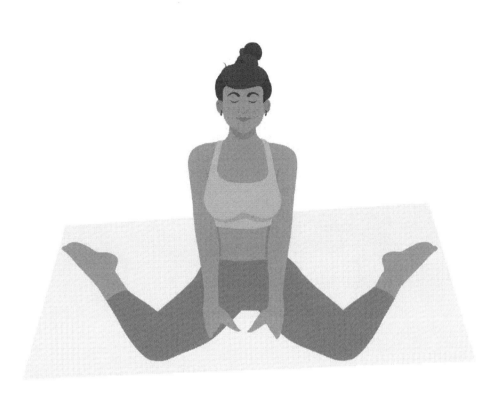

Bend between the ankles

Get on your knees, pull your buttocks back and sit between your ankles, leaving your feet on the sides of your buttocks. Calmly slowly descend to the ground until you bring yourself in extension with your back, shoulders, head and arms. If you can't, just simply sit betwcen your feet. Or you can get off and initially rest on your forearms. It remains for 30 to 60 seconds. Repeat the position twice.

Exercise 12

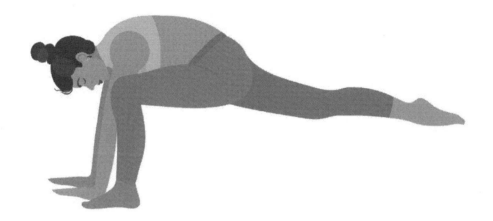

Bend your leg forward and bring your knee 90 degrees. Extend and straighten your back leg. Pull your chest forward, bring your hands to the ground and your heel up towards the ceiling. Bring your neck and back aligned with your hip. Stay 30 to 60 seconds repeat on the opposite side. Do the pose 2 times.

Back stretch

Back stretching exercises help improve posture and relieve joint and muscle pain. These exercises help prevent and improve sciatica and back pain.

Exercise 13

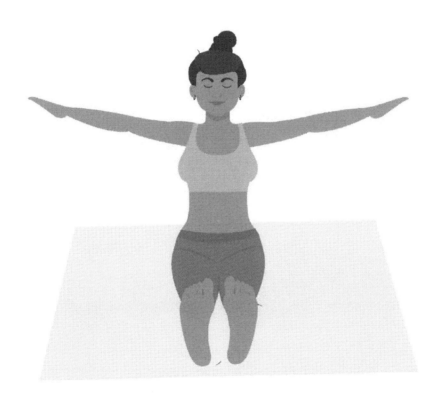

Sit on the ground with your feet stretched out in front of you. Bring your wrists under your shoulders and straighten your arms. Extend the column and bring yourself as straight as you can. Breathe slowly and stay for 30 to 60 seconds. Repeat 2 times.

Exercise 14

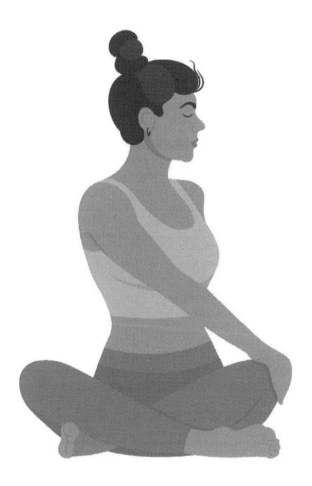

Sit comfortably, bend your leg and bring your right foot next to your left hip, cross your left leg over the leg that is resting on the ground. Bring your right arm in front of the crossed leg, oppose a slight tension. Rotate your torso slowly and bring your left arm behind your back. Stay in position for 30 to 60 seconds and repeat on the opposite side. Do the sequence 2 times.

Exercise 15

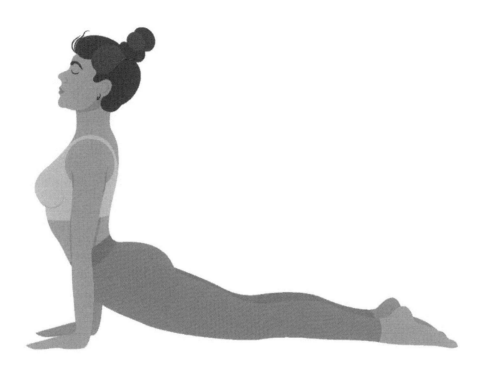

Lie on your stomach, with your palms resting on the ground, extend your arms and lift the trunk. Stay with your feet and shins on the floor, look forward and extend your back. Stay in position for 30 to 60 seconds. Perform the sequence 2 times.

Exercise 16

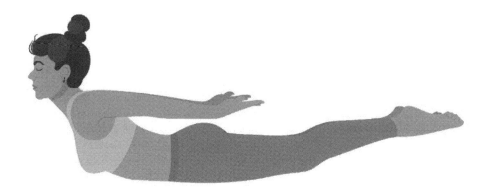

Lie on your stomach with your arms at your sides, bring your palms up. Simultaneously lifts shoulders, chest, head and legs. Don't flex your head, look ahead. Stay in this position for 20 seconds, repeat 3 times.

DON'T IN THE PRACTICE OF STRETCHING

Stretching can be adapted to everyone's physical needs, but it must be performed at suitable times and with suitable methods, without ever exaggerating. However, it can be contraindicated if it is practiced with forced movements: remember that the positions must not cause pain when reaching the full range of motion.

If you have suffered trauma, injuries to muscles, tendons, ligaments or joints, or in the presence of major diseases, always seek the advice of a specialist before practicing stretching.

A flexible body stays young longer. Perseverance and patience will lead your body to achieve excellent results.

6 SIMPLE EXERCISES TO PREPARE FOR A WALK

Before a good hike in the mountains, it is important to do some warm-up exercises. Here are 6 simple exercises to get you started on your hike.

Before a good hike in the mountains, it is important to do some warm-up exercises that often, however, due to laziness and lack of time, are not taken into consideration. Even if walking, in itself, is already a good warm-up for many sports, it is important to know that an excursion in the mountains requires much more effort than a simple walk, especially if the path has uphill sections (and in the mountains, you know, it is practically impossible to find totally flat itineraries) and if we have a backpack on our shoulders.

For this reason, it is essential to carry out exercises to help muscles, tendons and joints to be more fluid and flexible in view of the efforts to which they will be subjected. In reality, to do the warm-up exercises well, do not take more than 10 - 15 minutes, a truly negligible commitment when compared to the numerous benefits that are received. A well-performed warm-up, in fact, reduces fatigue, the onset of cramps, the risk of muscle and joint trauma and the classic sensation of sore legs in the days following the trip.

Here are 6 simple warm-up exercises to tackle your hike in the best way, starting from the ankles up to the shoulders and neck.

1- Ankles

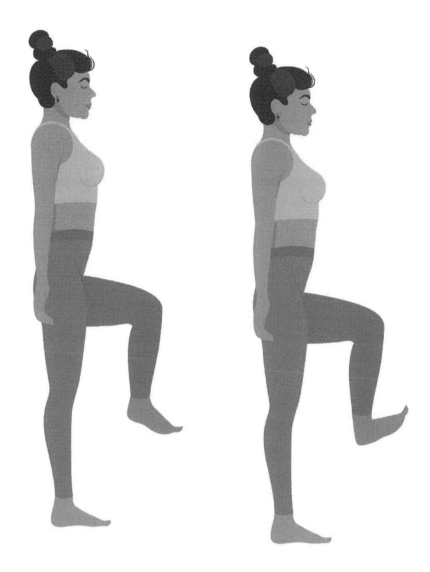

The ankles are essential because they allow both to unload the weight of the body to the ground and to make the foot perform all the fundamental movements to be able to walk, run, climb or descend stairs. Before a hike in the mountains, you need to prepare your ankles, simply by lifting first one foot and then the other from the ground and, in turn, first rotate them clockwise and counterclockwise and then up and down.

2- Calves

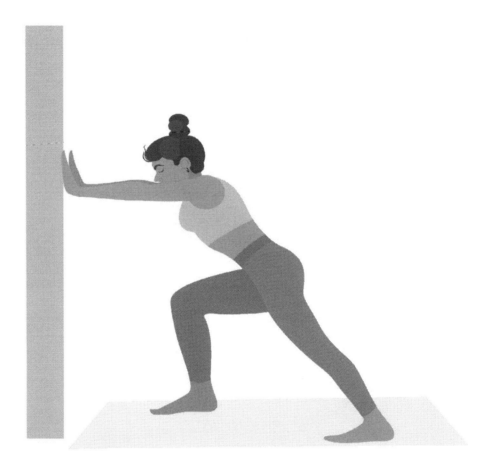

The calves are subjected to frequent changes in intensity and effort while trekking. You can warm up your calves by first doing tip-toe lifts and then stretching them. To stretch, stand in front of a wall, stretch your arms horizontally at shoulder height, resting your palms against the wall, and bring one leg back. Move your torso forward until you begin to feel the calf muscle pulling. Repeat the movement changing the position of the legs.

3- Knees

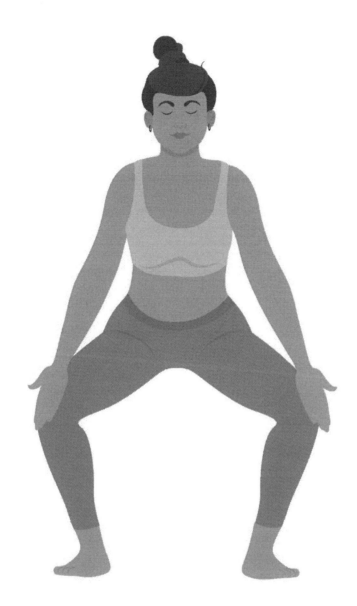

The descent represents the number one enemy of the knees which, in fact, often complain after long downhill stretches. This is why it is important to have adequate warm-up before walking, thus limiting inflammation of the ligaments. To prepare yourself better, bend your legs slightly, place your hands on your knees and perform rotational movements from the inside out and vice versa.

4- Quadriceps

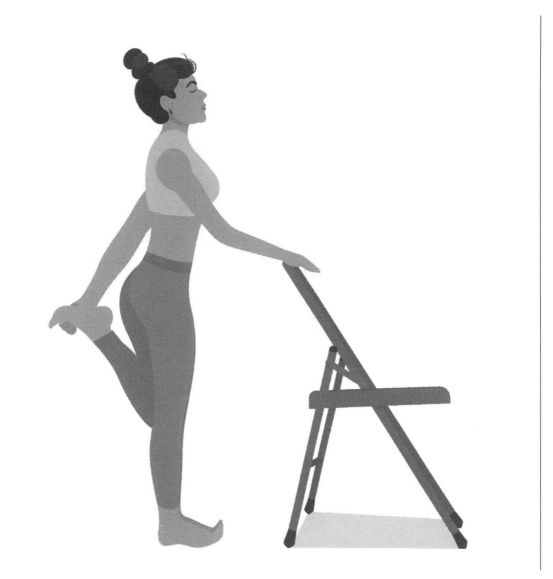

During walking, one of the most stressed muscles is the one located in the front of the thigh, that is the quadriceps, which helps to maintain balance and the knees movements. To warm up the quadriceps, stand up looking for support for one hand. Lift one leg by grabbing the ankle with one hand and bend it backwards until you feel tension in the muscle. Try to maintain an upright posture and avoid torso swaying.

5- Femoral biceps

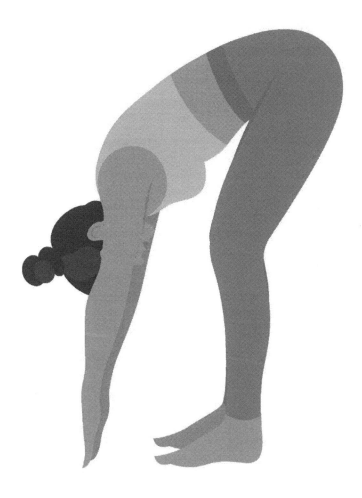

The hamstrings are the hamstrings, and in combination with the quadriceps, they help bend or flex the knees. While walking, the hamstrings are particularly stressed, much more so than during a run. To warm up your hamstrings, stand with your legs straight and knees together. Then bend your torso forward leaving your arms dangling and avoiding swaying or sudden movements.

6- Shoulders and neck

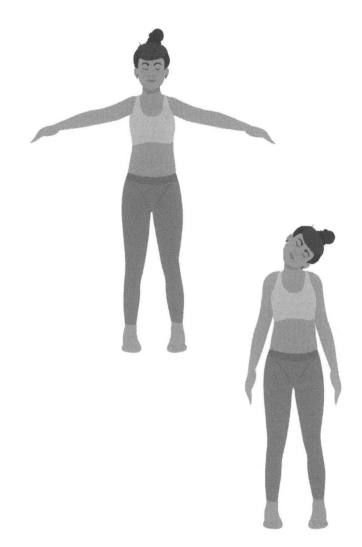

Now let's move on to the upper body, no less important than everything else. Even the shoulders and neck, in fact, play a fundamental role in maintaining posture and can be very stressed by the weight of the backpack. Start warming up your shoulders by doing simple arm circles. To relax the neck muscles, instead, perform rotations and bending of the head with slow and gentle movements.

Remember to maintain the positions for no more than 20/30 seconds and repeat the exercises two or three times very slowly, stopping as soon as you feel muscle fatigue: it is bad, in fact, to get out of breath (better to keep your breath for later!)

Physical exercises and stretching to combine with walking

Walking is good, but to prevent pain and trauma you also need to do physical exercises and stretching to strengthen bones, muscles and joints.

Walking is one of the simplest motor activities to carry out, because no particular skills or motor patterns are required, and you don't need to be an expert. We all know how to walk, because it is a motor action that we perform from early childhood. Walking is suitable for all fitness levels; you can do it anywhere. With walking you can have many benefits for heart health, for the respiratory system, for the mind and for weight loss but; if you want to strengthen the various muscle groups and prevent and relieve joint pain, in addition to walking you must also perform physical exercises.

WALKING AS A WORKOUT

When walking can be considered a workout and what its benefits are

To make a simple walk a workout, just walk at a faster, steadier pace. You must feel the heartbeat slightly faster than when just walking, the breath more intense, and your body warming up until you feel the sweat running down your back. If you feel all of this, it means that you are well on your way to turning a simple walk into a workout.

Walking at a more intense and faster pace can reduce the risk of heart disease, the risk of high cholesterol, high blood pressure and diabetes. Brisk walking helps improve sleep quality and reduces stress. This type of moderate exercise helps you maintain optimal long-term health and control your body weight.

Why is it necessary, in addition to brisk walking, to perform physical exercises and stretching to keep muscles, bones healthy and relieve pain?

Brisk walking is one of the medium-intense aerobic activities, so it only provides a number of benefits. To obtain other benefits for bones, muscles, tendons and ligaments, a series of exercises must also be combined with walking, to improve strength, endurance, balance and flexibility. Try these simple exercises.

5 dynamic stretching exercises to be performed before a walk

Dynamic stretching can be done before any training routine. It helps warm up the body and prepare the muscles to work, which can improve performance and reduce the risk of injury. Do these exercises before a brisk walk.

PELVIS SURROUND:

stand with your heels as wide as your hips. Make 10 circles with your pelvis clockwise and 10 anti-clockwise.

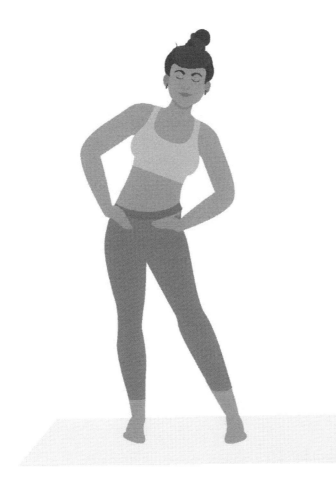

SIDE LEG OPENING:

stand upright, hold on to a wall for support if you don't have good balance. Raise and lower your right leg sideways without resting your foot on the ground. Complete 15 reps and then switch legs.

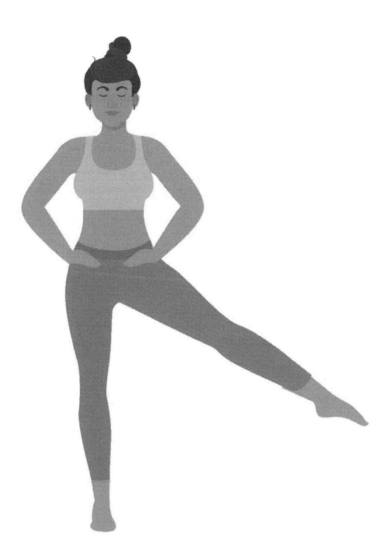

HIGH KNEE WALK:

stand up straight, bend and lift first the right knee and then the left as high as possible alternately. Do 20 repetitions.

Keep your back straight as you lift your knees.

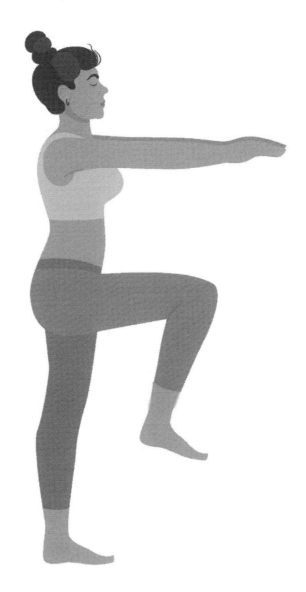

WALK IN PLACE BACK AND FORTH:

stand up straight and keep your feet hip-width apart. Take one step forward and one back with the right foot without lifting the left heel off the floor, repeat for 30 seconds, first with the right foot and then with the left one.

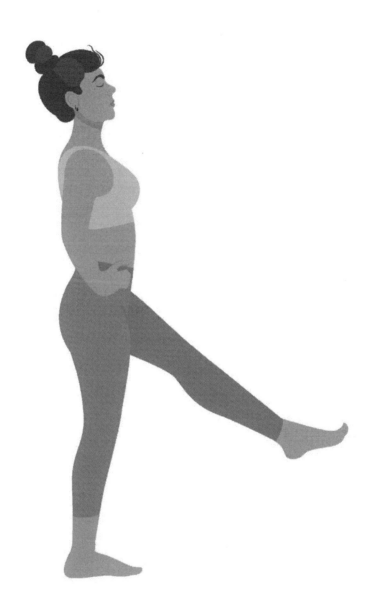

BALLERINA HALF SQUAT:

stand with your heels wider than your hips and your toes slightly aiming outward. Lift your heels as high as you can, hold for 3 seconds, bring your heels back to the ground, push your hips back, bend your knees and do a half squat. Repeat 15 times.

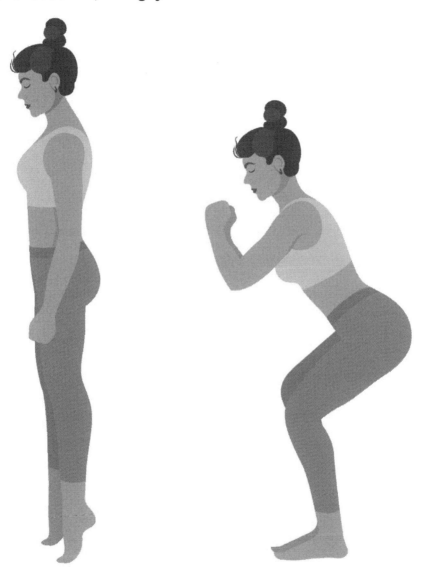

Lose weight while walking: here is the effective training program.

3 exercises to strengthen the arms

Do these exercises before or after the walk or on days when you don't do the brisk walk.

HIGH PLANK:

get into a high plank position, keep a straight line from head to toe with your palms flat on the ground, arms and legs outstretched. Activate the core and stay for 30 seconds. Repeat 2 times.

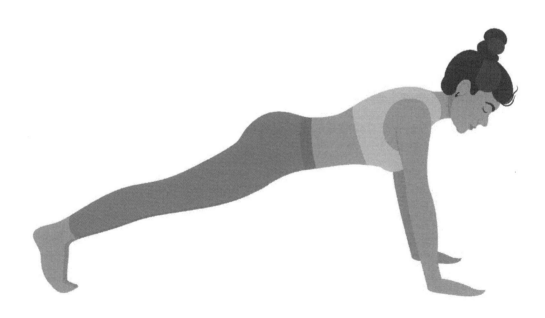

DIP TO SHELF:

sit on the edge of a chair or bench. Grab the forward edge of the chair with your hands, lift your buttocks forward out of the chair. Then bend and straighten your arms, without moving your back too far from the edge of the seat of the chair as you go up and down with your arms. Do 10-20 repetitions 2 times.

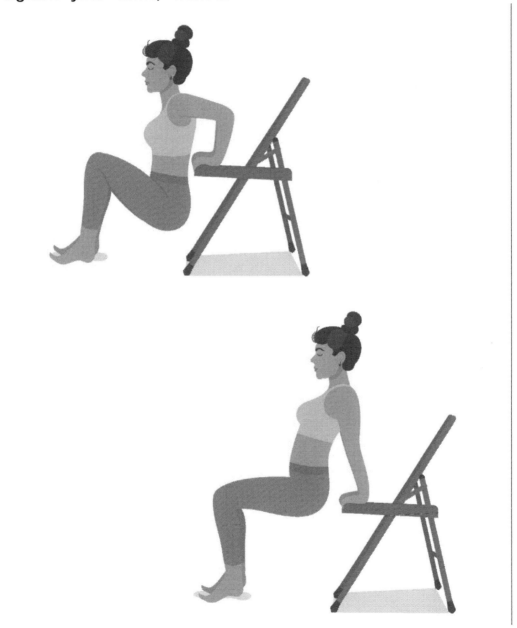

ARM WRAPPING:

stand with your back straight and open your arms in a cross. Keep your elbows slightly bent and your wrists on the shoulder line. Perform 20 clockwise and 20 anti-clockwise circles. If you want to intensify the exercise, hold small weights or 2 bottles of water in your hands.

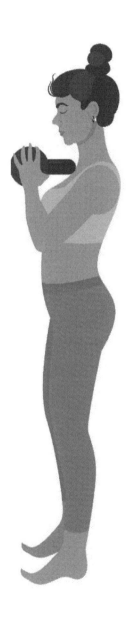

3 exercises to strengthen the back

Do these exercises before or after the walk or on days when you don't do the brisk walk.

BRIDGE:

lie with your back on the ground and your hands at your sides, legs bent, and keep your feet flat on the ground. Lift your hips off the ground, squeeze your buttocks and stay there 5 seconds. Slowly lower your hips without touching the floor. Do 20 repetitions, 2 times.

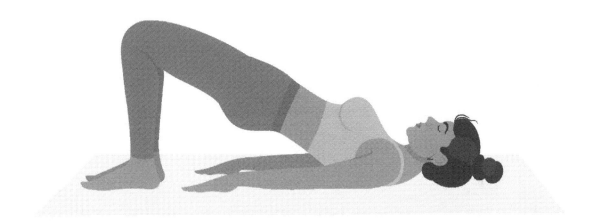

CAT-COW: on all 4 limbs.

Keep your shoulders above your wrists and knees as wide as your hips. Exhale, push the pubis forward and the coccyx down as if to close the navel. Inhale, arch your back and push the tailbone up as if to open the navel.

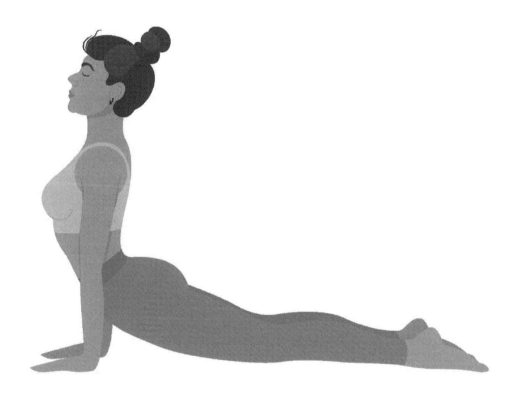

COBRA:

- lie on your stomach with your palms close to your shoulders.
- Lift your torso, pushing on your hands, and leave your knees and feet on the ground.
- Lift and arch your torso as you straighten your arms without feeling discomfort in your lower back.

- Arch your back and straighten your arms according to your fitness level.
- For easier execution place 2 pillows under the pubis. Using the pillows will help you straighten your arms and arch your back better.

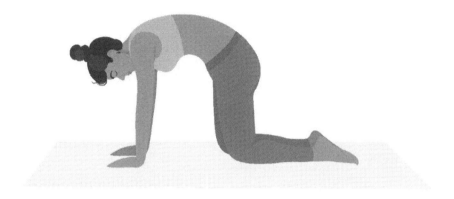

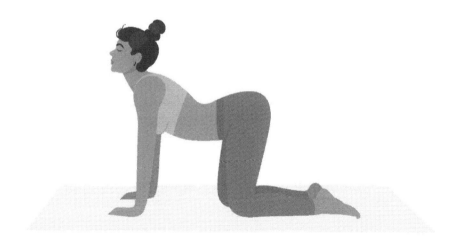

5 static stretching exercises to do after walking

Static stretching involves stretching a muscle or joint. Certain positions are taken and held for a set period of time. For example, if you reach out to touch your toes, once you have stretched as much as possible, you must maintain the stretch position for a set duration.

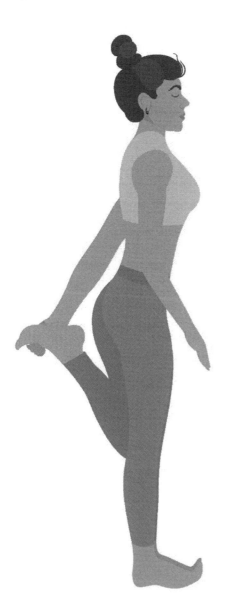

QUADRICEPS HAMSTRING STRETCH: **stand up straight and pull a leg behind you with the corresponding hand. Try to bring the heel towards the buttock. Keep your knee pointing down as you perform this stretch to protect the knee joint. Press and hold your heel behind your thigh for at least 30 seconds, then switch sides.**

POSTERIOR THIGH STRETCH:

- sit on the ground and extend your left leg.
- Move the right foot towards the inside of the left thigh, so that the sole of the foot touches the inside of the thigh, if possible.
- Extend your hands forward to reach your left foot.
- Bend over but without rounding your back.
- Hold the position for at least 30 seconds. Repeat with the other leg.

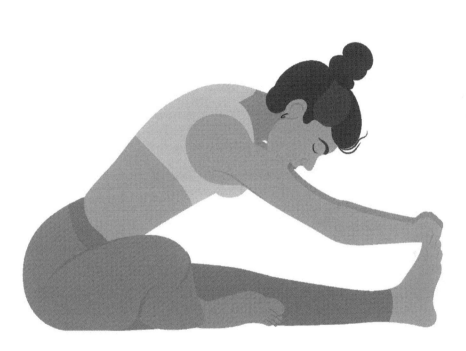

PIRIFORMIS AND GLUTE STRETCH:

- lie on your back with your knees bent and feet flat on the floor.
- Cross your right ankle over your left knee.
- Grab the back of your left thigh with your hands and bring your leg towards your chest.
- Hold for at least 30 seconds, then switch sides. You should feel the stretch in the back of the thigh and buttocks.

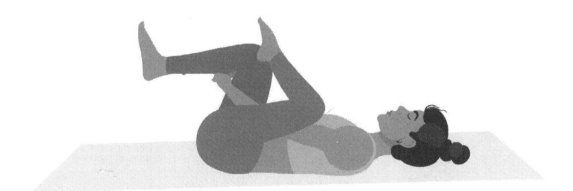

LUMBAR STRETCH:

- lie on your back.
- Grab both knees and pull them towards your chest.

- Hold the position for 30 seconds.

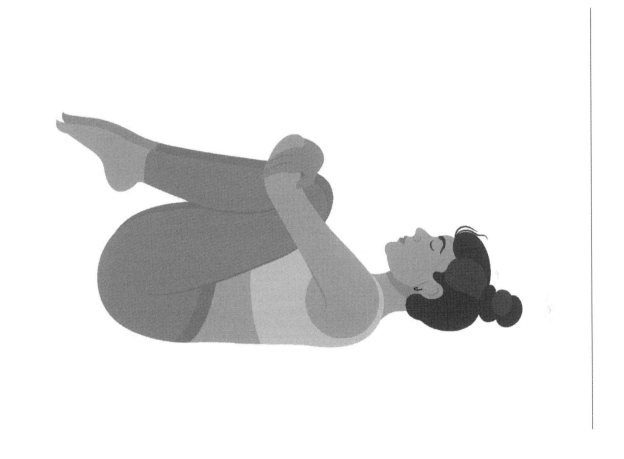

LEGS AGAINST A WALL:

lie on your back and raise your legs high against a wall for 2 minutes.

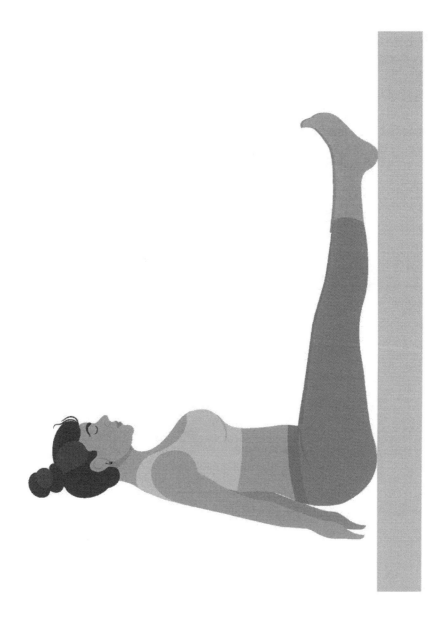

Do these exercises every time you go for a walk or even at other times of the day at least 2-3 times a week.

Exercises to improve balance

In order for our body to be in balance, the inner ear and eyes continuously record our position in space. With the brain and muscles we therefore constantly correct our position, keeping us upright and we do this without having to concentrate.

So why train your balance?

Even if maintaining balance happens unconsciously, it is worth training it, because just like muscle strength, we can improve it in a targeted way. When muscles are prepared for these situations, they react more effectively and protect us, for example, from exaggerated reactions such as sprains.

What may seem abstract is visible on the tightrope: if you first step on a tightrope with one foot, the leg shakes and the rope wobbles back and forth. The muscles react too strongly and too late on both sides. With a little exercise, the muscles will work more efficiently and only minor corrections will be needed to keep the body in balance.

For whom is balance training particularly suitable?

The answer is: for everyone! Especially with age, we often move less and the risk of falling increases. The sooner you start to train your balance the better, since well-exercised balance with fast muscles is the best prevention against falls.

Exercise 1: Stand on one leg

Bend one leg forward or backward and remain standing on the other leg for as long as possible.

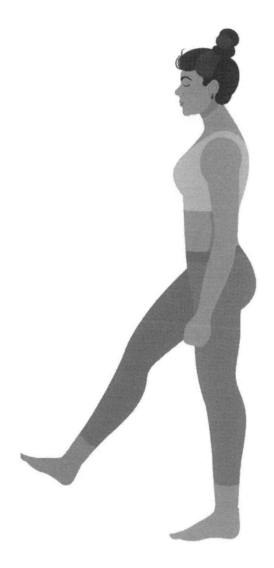

To make it more difficult:

- Move the bent leg alternately forwards and backwards
- Close your eyes
- Tilt your head back
- Tilt your head back with your eyes closed

Exercise 2: Standing position with feet aligned

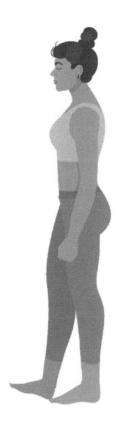

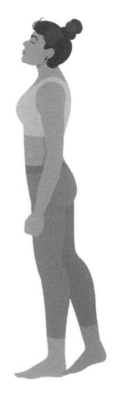

Place one foot in front of the foot on which your weight rests. The heel of the front foot touches the toes of the rear foot. Hold the position as long as possible.

So, it becomes more difficult:

- Close your eyes
- Tilt your head back
- Tilt your head back with your eyes closed
- Place your foot behind the foot on which the weight rests

Exercise 3: Stand on your toes

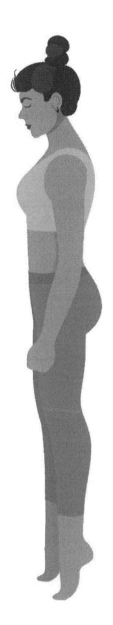

Stand with both feet on your toes. Maintain the position for as long as possible.

To make it more difficult:

- Spring up by lowering and raising your heels.
- Tiptoe on one leg
- Stand with one leg on tiptoe on a rolled-up pillow or blanket

Exercise 4: Raise the leg to the side

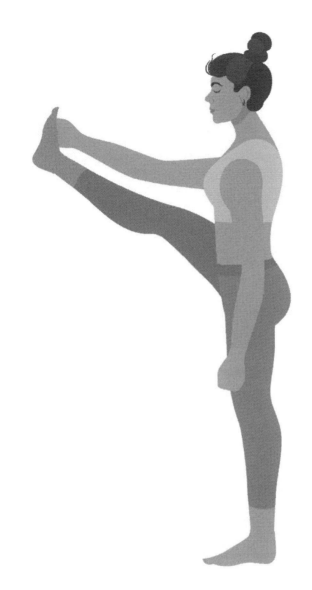

Stand on one leg and lift the other leg sideways as much as possible, keeping the torso always in an upright position.

So, it becomes more difficult:

- Move the raised leg forward, sideways and backward without touching the ground
- Do the same thing with your eyes closed

Exercise 5: Lunge

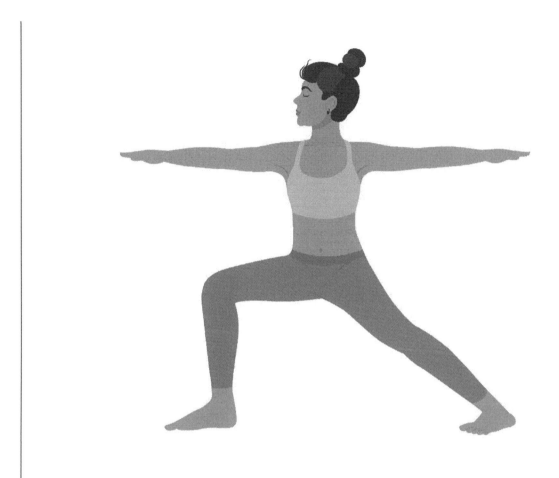

Step forward with one leg, step back with the other leg. Lower the pelvis until the knee of the front leg forms a right angle. Straighten up and repeat the exercise.

So, it becomes more difficult:

- Place your front foot, back foot, or both feet on a pillow or rolled blanket
- Decrease the distance between the feet
- Close your eyes

How to train the pelvic floor

Taking care of the pelvic floor, a muscular structure connected to sphincter control and sexual well-being, is an important gesture of love and attention to one's body, especially for women, and can be done through simple exercises.

WHAT IS THE PELVIC FLOOR?

The structure of the pelvic floor forms the basis of the group of muscles responsible for maintaining the so-called core, that is, the central area of the body that favors lumbo-pelvic stability and allows the whole body to be strong.

The pelvic floor is made up of layers of muscles and other connective tissues. These muscle bands extend just like an imaginary hammock, from the pubis to the coccyx and from one ischial tuberosity (to be clear, the bony protrusions that are perceived on the buttocks when sitting) to the other.

This important structure works with the diaphragm and with the deep muscles of the abdomen and back to support the spine and control the pressure inside the abdomen.

The pelvic floor muscles also support the bladder, intestines and, in women, the uterus. They prevent urinary and fecal incontinence, in addition to prolapses, and are important for the well-being of the sexual and reproductive sphere.

RISK FACTORS FOR THE HEALTH OF THE PELVIC FLOOR

The pelvic floor can be weakened by pregnancy, childbirth, prostate cancer treatment, obesity and muscle strain caused by chronic constipation or certain sports.

Poor posture, while walking or sitting (for example standing for many hours with your back leaning forward or with your legs crossed), can also lead to deterioration in pelvic floor health.

Let's now go into the specifics of the most frequent risk factors and give some useful information on the importance of this muscle structure not only for women, but also for men.

The muscles in this area can also be compromised by some sports.

What makes certain sports disciplines enemies of the pelvic floor are the constant shocks, rubbing, contractures and stresses to which these muscles are subjected during practice.

In particular, the sports that most of all have a negative impact on pelvic floor health are:

- spinning;
- horse riding;
- skiing;
- dance (both classical and modern);
- crossfit;
- weights.

Physical activities such as fitness, walking and yoga, on the other hand, do not present particular contraindications, if carried out correctly. Yoga is even recommended for women who wish to improve pelvic floor health and gain greater awareness of this part of the body.

Pregnancy

There are several factors that can affect the health of the pelvic floor during a pregnancy, from the weight of the uterus to the muscular efforts to which this area is subjected during the expulsive phase of childbirth.

In the presence of an untrained pelvic floor, any lacerations and weakening of the muscle structure can unfortunately cause more intense and permanent damage.

The importance of the pelvic floor also for men

Good pelvic floor health affects not only women, but men as well.

As for men, the pelvic floor muscles also support the bladder and intestines in the male body. The openings of these organs (the urethra for the bladder and the rectum for the intestine) pass through the pelvic muscles.

Hence, even in a man the presence of strong pelvic floor muscles helps prevent the uncontrolled leakage of urine and feces, and supports sexual functions.

HOW TO ASSESS THE HEALTH OF THE PELVIC FLOOR

It is not always easy to detect the symptoms of any pelvic floor problems, but now that we have studied the location and importance of this muscle structure, it may be easier to understand if certain problems are related to a weakening or hypertonicity of the pelvic muscles.

The most common symptoms of pelvic floor dysfunction are:

Incontinence: urinary or fecal;

Sphincter problems: difficulty in urinating, haemorrhoids, pelvic weight sensation, constipation;

Sexual problems: pain during intercourse, difficulty in reaching orgasm, impotence, etc.

The occurrence of one or more of these symptoms, especially in association with the risk factors we have already talked about, can indicate the presence of pelvic problems.

HOW IS THE PELVIC FLOOR ASSESSMENT PERFORMED?

If a woman suffers from the symptoms, it is erroneously thought that, given the location and functions of these muscle groups, the most suitable doctor to contact for an evaluation of the pelvic floor is the trusted gynecologist.

In reality, a gynecologist does not necessarily know how to carry out a thorough and timely evaluation of the pelvic floor: to be able to do this, you must have followed specific refresher courses on the subject.

This is why even figures such as the midwife or the surgeon specializing in coloproctology, if qualified and enabled, can examine the correct functioning of these muscles.

The latter specialist represents, together with the urologist, the reference figure for men who wish to deepen the health of their pelvic floor.

The evaluation of the pelvic muscles takes place with manual exploration of the vagina and / or rectum. Having to test the muscle tone of the bands present in this internal area of the body, it will be necessary to introduce a finger into the vagina and / or anus, asking the patient to breathe and voluntarily contractions in order to effectively evaluate the stability and strength of the muscles.

HOW TO TRAIN THE PELVIC FLOOR?

To exercise the pelvic floor in the correct way, it is important to first identify the muscles to be toned, so as not to make mistakes and exercise other muscle groups.

It is not always easy to find the pelvic floor muscles. To locate them, it may be helpful to follow these steps:

Sit comfortably with your knees slightly apart. Imagine having to hold back flatulence, thus contracting the muscles normally responsible for this action. But the buttocks and legs shouldn't move at all.

Now imagine urinating and blocking the flow of urine. You should use the same group of muscles that you solicited before, but you will seem to be able to control the impulse with more force (be careful, however, never to block urine during urination, because it could cause bladder problems).

Try to tighten the muscles around the anus, vagina and perineum, as if trying to block the passage of gas and urine at the same time. The first few times you will probably also contract muscles that do not concern the pelvic floor: the goal of the exercises we suggest is to try to isolate the affected muscle groups as much as possible without squeezing the legs and above all without contracting the buttocks or stopping breathing.

As soon as you feel able to identify your pelvic floor muscles, you can try the following exercises:

Exercise 1

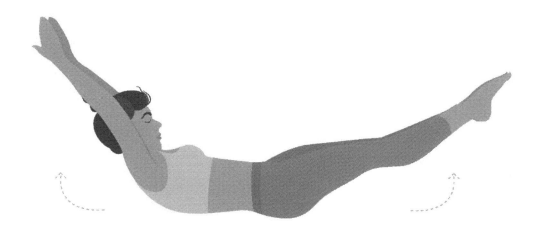

- Sit, or stand or lie down, with your knees slightly apart;
- Slowly squeeze and contract the muscles with enough force to keep them in tension for as long as possible (10 seconds, for example); release and rest for 4 seconds;
- Resume the contraction of the muscles, being careful to train the pelvic floor muscles and not others.

Since the goal of these exercises is also to make the pelvic muscles more resistant to sudden stress or strain, such as a laugh or a cough, it is possible to try this variant of the previous workout:

Exercise 2

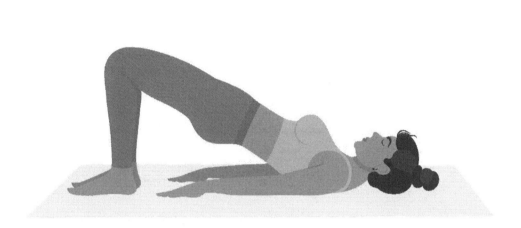

- Get into a lying, sitting or standing position, with your legs slightly apart;
- Identify the pelvic floor muscles;
- Contract and relax the muscles at quick intervals.
- The ideal is to do both sets of exercises 3-4 times a day, one after the other.

Exercises for back pain

The first exercise for back pain is to strive to listen to common sense by consulting a doctor before starting workouts. This is a real recommendation, designed to ensure that there are no contraindications to sports.

The exercises proposed in this chapter represent a general indication useful only for cases of back pain due to weakness or excessive muscle contractures (where back pain is a consequence of herniated discs, protrusions or other problems with the intervertebral discs, it is essential to contact an expert doctor and follow his instructions).

Often, those who follow a specific program to improve back health do not give the right importance to stretching exercises. This is most likely due to the fact that these stretching exercises constitute the final part of the session, thus resulting, erroneously, a physical activity of the session of secondary importance.

In fact, the role of these exercises is nothing short of fundamental. In fact, to prevent back pain, it is important to regain lost elasticity without limiting attention to just improving muscle strength. This type of training allows you to relieve tension and improve the elasticity of the paravertebral and lumbar muscles. Especially in the first period, when the inflammation and pain have not yet completely resolved, physical activity should be based almost exclusively on decompression exercises of the spine.

The proposed exercises do not require special tools and can be performed both in the gym and at home.

Exercise 1

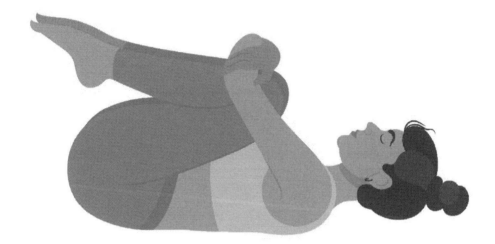

- Lie on the ground on your back;
- Bring your knees to your chest by bringing them as close as possible, with the help of your arms;

- Hold the position for 20 seconds, relax for a few seconds and repeat two more times.

Exercise 2

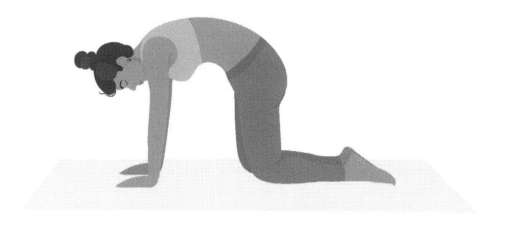

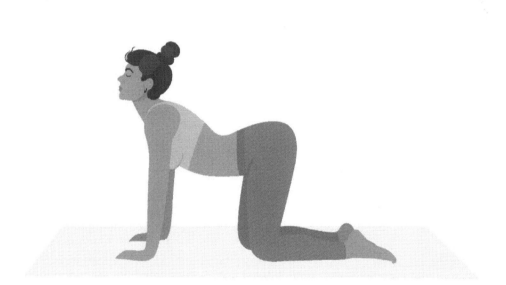

- On all fours on the ground (kneel, place your hands forward resting them on the floor shoulder-width apart);
- Breathe out by curving the spine upwards until the lungs are completely empty;
- While inhaling, slowly return to the starting position by flattening your back;
- Repeat 5 times.

Exercise 3

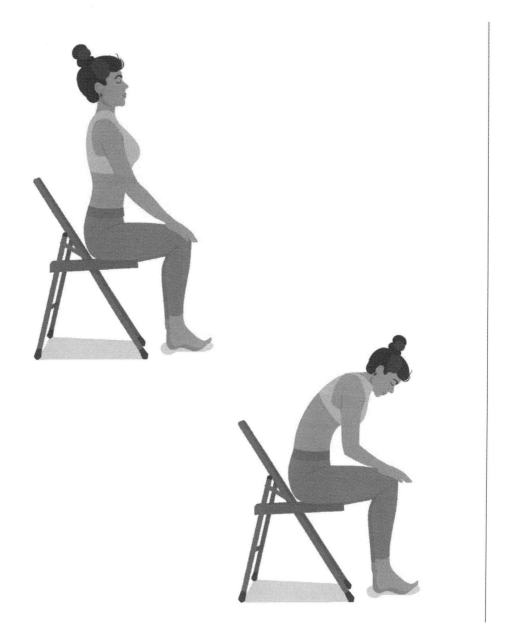

- Sit in a chair with your legs apart;
- As you exhale, bend your torso forward;
- While inhaling, slowly return to the starting position;
- Repeat 5 times.

Exercise 4

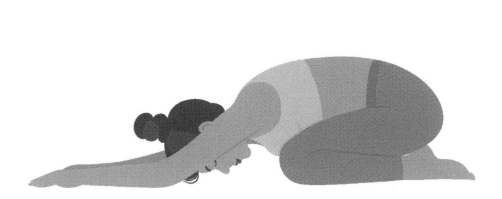

- Kneel on the ground, with your buttocks resting on your heels;
- As you exhale, bring your arms forward while keeping your pelvis in the starting position;
- While inhaling, slowly return to the starting position;
- Repeat by stretching your arms first to the right and then to the left.

Exercise 5

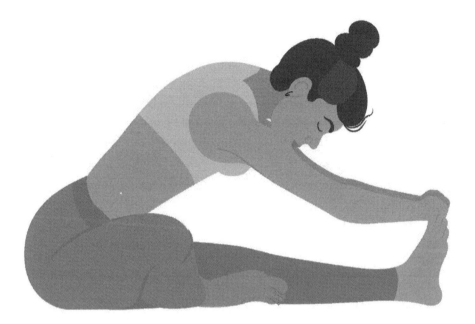

- Sitting on the ground, extend one leg and flex the other so that the sole of the foot is in contact with the inner part of the extended thigh;

- Extend both arms and torso forward so as to bring the toes closer to the tip of the foot;
- Hold the position for about 20 mins, then slowly return to the starting position and repeat for the other side.

Exercise 6

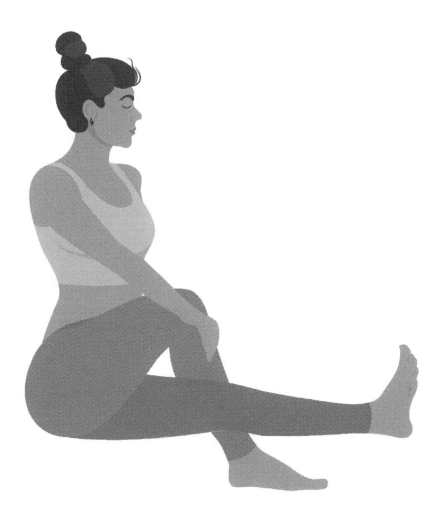

- Seated, one leg extended, the other crossed over the first;
- With the contralateral elbow, push the bent leg inwards by rotating the torso and head in the opposite direction;
- Hold the position for 15-20 seconds and repeat for the opposite side.

Exercise 7

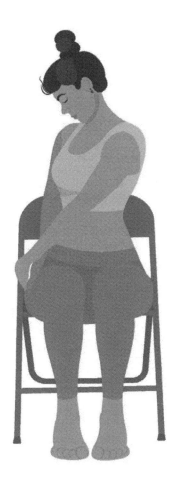

- While standing or sitting, slowly flex your neck to the side;
- With the hand on the side towards which the neck is bent, grasp the wrist of the opposite arm and pull it slightly downwards to tension the contralateral trapezius and shoulder muscles;
- Hold the position for 20-30 seconds and switch sides.

Always perform a general warm-up before starting any stretching exercises; wear comfortable clothing that does not impede movement; choose a relaxing environment and respect the correct breathing technique; avoid sudden movements and excessive stretching.

Conclusions

Older people can perform specific exercises to strengthen the abdominals and other stabilizing muscles of the trunk and pelvis in order to improve their body balance.

This translates into a better protective function of the spine, an improvement in posture and a greater ability to perform more or less complex movements both during sports and in everyday life.

For this purpose, we have created a real Core Training, four simple and effective exercises to train the core muscles or the main stabilizing muscles of the pelvis and trunk, including the abdominals (rectus abdominis, obliques and transverse).

Good joint stability allows for adequate motor control and optimal force application during daily activities such as climbing or descending stairs, picking up an object from the ground, ironing, etc.

In short, core stability exercises serve to:

- *Strengthen the abdomen, buttocks and back.*
- *Improve balance (hence the name, core stability).*
- *Prevent back pain and injuries even in old age.*

However, it is good practice to consult your doctor before performing the exercises listed below.

Lateral leg raises

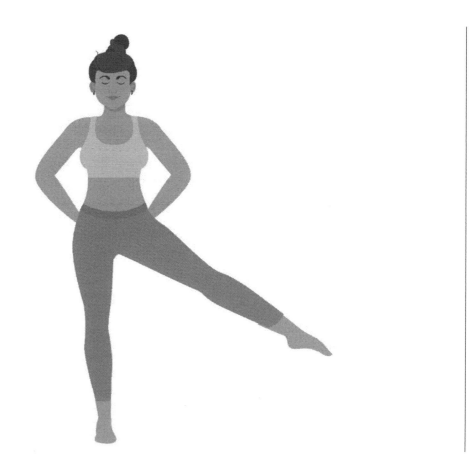

REPS: **10 per leg**

SERIES: **1-3**

INTENSITY: **light to moderate**

TIME: **2 mins**

REST PERIOD: **30-90 seconds between sets**

STARTING POSITION: **standing erect with feet together and hands on hips.**

EXECUTION: **exhale as you lift your left leg to the side and then return to the starting position. Keep the trunk and shoulders aligned throughout the movement by contracting the abdomen. Perform all repetitions, then repeat with the right leg.**

TIPS:

Maintain the curves of the spine.

Stabilize the supporting leg by contracting the buttocks and abdomen.

Front legs raise

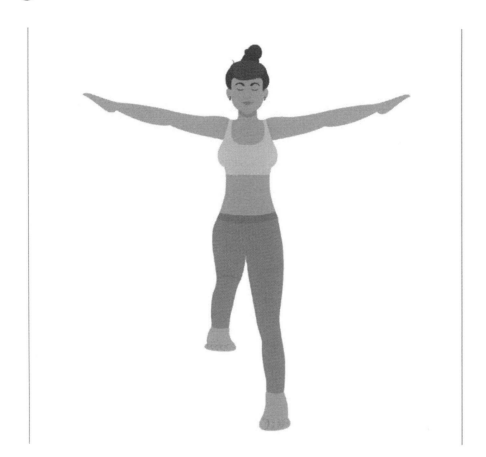

REPS: **10 per leg**

SERIES: **1-3**

INTENSITY: **light to moderate**

TIME: **2 mins**

REST PERIOD: **30-90 seconds between sets**

STARTING POSITION: **Stand with feet together. Arms at your sides for balance.**

EXECUTION: **lift the right knee up as far as possible, then lower the foot to the ground. Perform all repetitions, then repeat with the left leg.**

TIPS:

Maintain the curves of the spine.

Stabilize the supporting leg by contracting the buttocks and abdomen.

Half lunges

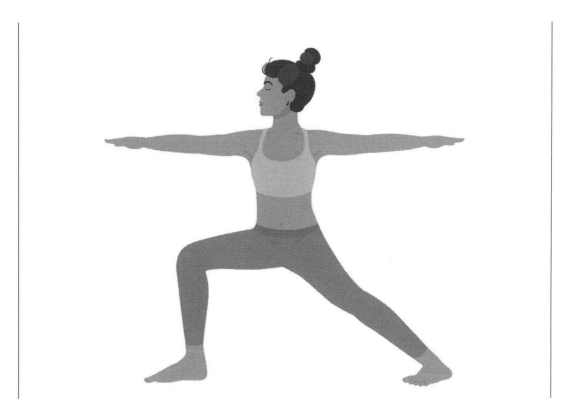

REPS: **10**

SERIES: **1-3**

INTENSITY: **moderate to high**

TIME: **2 mins**

REST PERIOD: **30-90 seconds between sets**

STARTING POSITION: **Stand with feet together. Arms at your sides for balance.**

EXECUTION: **take a step forward and bend the left leg almost to form a right** angle. The leg to be bent is the left, so the right leg flexes accordingly, not the other way around.

Return to the starting position and repeat the same movement with the right leg.

TIPS AND TECHNIQUES:

Distribute your body weight evenly between the right and left foot.

In the lunge position, the back shoulder, hip and knee should be aligned.

Half squats

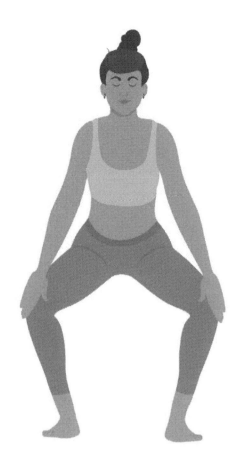

REPS: **10**

SERIES: **1-3**

INTENSITY: **moderate**

TIME: **2 mins**

REST PERIOD: **30-90 seconds between sets**

STARTING POSITION: **Standing with legs apart with feet in slight external rotation and hands resting on the thighs.**

EXECUTION: **bend your knees slightly while keeping your back straight. Stop before the buttocks reach the level of the knees. Exhale as you return to the starting position.**

TIPS:

Do not lift your heels off the ground.

Contract the abdominal and gluteal muscles throughout the entire range of motion.

References

1   https://www.slideshare.net/hassanfaizan4/hyperbolic-stretchingpdf-251993336

2   https://www.popsugar.com/fitness/Body-Weight-Exercises-34376556

3 https://www.nuvovivo.com/blog/exercises-to-relieve-your-back-pain/

4   https://www.livestrong.com/article/13767831-get-up-exercises/

5 https://evelo.com/blogs/learn/exercise-guide-for-seniors

6 https://www.ncbi.nlm.nih.gov/pmc/articles/PMC8704638/

7   https://www.livestrong.com/article/106917-core-strengthening-exercises-seniors/

8   https://www.frontiersin.org/articles/10.3389/fphys.2022.796097/full

9   https://samarpanphysioclinic.com/lower-back-strengthening-exercises/

10 https://www.getpersonalgrowth.com/en/crunch-a-terra

11   https://www.healthline.com/health/exercise-fitness/muscle-groups-to-workout-together

12 https://www.healthline.com/health/core-strength-more-important-than-muscular-arms

13 https://topfitnesshome.com/calf-pain-relief-exercises/

14   https://www.curves.eu/en/the-importance-of-reinforcing-the-upper-body/

15 https://en.wikipedia.org/wiki/Strength_training

16 https://www.gym-pact.com/russian-twist-alternative

17   https://www.foodspring.co.uk/magazine/breathing-while-lifting

18 https://bmcpublichealth.biomedcentral.com/articles/10.1186/s12889-021-10565-7

19   https://www.health.harvard.edu/staying-healthy/3-surprising-risks-of-poor-posture

20 https://health.clevelandclinic.org/health-effects-of-poor-posture/

21   https://blog.iafstore.com/en/ab-exercises-without-involving-the-iliopsoas-a284

22 https://www.wikihow.com/Do-Forward-Splits

23   https://www.slideshare.net/hassanfaizan4/hyperbolic-stretchingpdf-251993336#:~:text=Stretching is an

exercise technique that lengthens and, pain, brings the body towards complete physical well-being.

24 https://modern-women.net/20482779-physical-exercises-and-stretching-to-combine-with-walking

25   https://www.ncbi.nlm.nih.gov/pmc/articles/PMC3806175/

26   https://www.verywellfit.com/medicine-ball-exercises-1231106

27   https://www.healthline.com/health/fitness/superman-exercise

28   https://www.healthline.com/health/fitness/all-about-your-core-what-it-is-what-it-does-and-how-to-use-it

29   https://www.ncbi.nlm.nih.gov/pmc/articles/PMC7249999/

30   https://www.womenshealthmag.com/fitness/a20702682/wall-workout/

31 https://travelunziped.com/stretching-exercises/

32   https://www.betterhealth.vic.gov.au/health/conditionsandtreatments/abdominal-muscles#:~:text=Your core

muscles are the muscles deep within,of the pelvic floor, and the oblique muscles.

33   https://www.culturepartnership.eu/en/article/10-tips-for-successful-event

34 https://fitnessvolt.com/australian-pull-ups/

35 https://www.bodybuilding.com/exercises/russian-twist

36 https://orthophysio.com/know-your-injury/physiotherapy/stretching-myths-and-facts/

37 https://www.catalystathletics.com/article/49/The-Olympic-Lift-Starting-Position-Snatch-Clean/

38 https://www.healthline.com/health/fitness-exercise/benefits-of-aerobic-exercise

39 https://foodnhealth.org/5-reasons-important-strong-core-muscles/

40 https://link.springer.com/chapter/10.1007/978-3-030-54506-2_3

41 https://www.medicalnewstoday.com/articles/weak-hip-flexors-symptoms

42 https://www.stack.com/a/5-medicine-ball-exercise-for-developing-power/

43 https://bmcmusculoskeletdisord.biomedcentral.com/articles/10.1186/s12891-021-04858-6

44 https://www.bbc.co.uk/bitesize/guides/zhvv2sg/revision/4

45 https://wellbeingport.com/are-reverse-crunches-more-effective/

46 https://www.physio-pedia.com/Centre_of_Gravity

47 https://www.britannica.com/science/abdominal-muscle

48 https://www.physitrack.ca/exercise-library/how-to-perform-seated-calf-stretch

49 https://myhealth.alberta.ca/health/aftercareinformation/pages/conditions.aspx?hwid=bo1540

50 https://www.verywellfit.com/single-leg-stance-exercise-for-better-balance-2696233

51 https://en.wikipedia.org/wiki/Intermuscular_coordination#:~:text=Intermuscular coordination describes the

coordination within different muscles, joints, as well as stabilisation of body positioning.

52 https://www.wholelifechallenge.com/why-10-minutes-of-exercise-per-day-is-enough-to-get-you-results/

53 https://southvanphysio.com/why-is-core-stability-important/#:~:text=A healthy core is important in preventing

accidents, posture. It even assists with breathing and digestion.

54 https://forum.wordreference.com/threads/you-need-to-do-a-lot-of-practice.3117018/

55 https://healthy.kaiserpermanente.org/health-wellness/healtharticle.7-simple-exercises-you-can-do-at-home

56 https://www.nhlbi.nih.gov/health/lungs/body-controls-breathing

57 https://www.nhs.uk/Planners/pregnancycareplanner/Documents/BandBF_pelvic_floor_women.pdf

58 https://www.popworkouts.com/leg-lifts-exercise/

59 https://lifestyle.fit/en/training/fitness/russian-twists-muscles-benefits/

60 https://www.yogapoint.com/pranayama/types-of-pranayama.htm

61 https://www.physio-pedia.com/Quadriceps_Muscle

62 https://www.ncbi.nlm.nih.gov/pmc/articles/PMC4817590/

63 https://www.ncbi.nlm.nih.gov/books/NBK537056/

64 https://wjes.biomedcentral.com/articles/10.1186/s13017-018-0167-4

65 https://www.healthline.com/health/fitness-exercise/essential-runner-stretches

66 https://www.css.ch/en/private-customers/my-health/exercise/exercises/balance-exercises.html

67 https://www.ncbi.nlm.nih.gov/pmc/articles/PMC1472875/

68 https://www.maudmedical.com/research-education/pelvic-floor-muscles

69 https://www.setforset.com/blogs/news/core-stability-training-anti-rotational-vs-rotational-core-exercises

70   https://www.sportsmith.co/articles/what-do-activation-or-pre-activation-exercises-actually-do-anything/

71   https://workouttrends.com/how-to-do-superman-exercise

72   https://www.frontiersin.org/articles/10.3389/fphys.2022.813243/full

73   https://www.sweat.com/blogs/fitness/how-to-breathe-when-exercising#:~:text=When it comes to strength

training, exhaling as,starting position is most efficient and considered best-practice.

74   https://www.healthline.com/human-body-maps/diaphragm

75   https://www.sportswebsites.org/what-is-footwork-in-badminton-and-how-to-practice-in-the-right-way/

76   https://www.healthline.com/health/fitness-exercise/plank-exercise-benefits

77 https://en.wikipedia.org/wiki/Karate_stances

78   https://context.reverso.net/traduzione/inglese-italiano/tilt your head back

79

https://www.nhstaysidecdn.scot.nhs.uk/NHSTaysideWeb/idcplg?IdcService=GET_SECURE_FILE&dDocName=PR

OD_212453&Rendition=web&RevisionSelectionMethod=LatestReleased&noSaveAs=1#:~:text=Imagine that

you are trying to stop yourself, your breath, and to continue to breathe gently.

80   https://www.mayoclinic.org/healthy-lifestyle/womens-health/in-depth/kegel-exercises/art-20045283

81   https://www.greenactitude.com/en/abdominal-vacuum-a-simple-breathing-exercise-to-have-a-flat-stomach

82 https://pubmed.ncbi.nlm.nih.gov/29933200/

83 https://idioms.thefreedictionary.com/be well on your way to

84 https://buddingoptimist.com/ways-to-exercise/

85 https://breathe.ersjournals.com/content/14/2/166

Made in the USA
Columbia, SC
20 May 2024